# PSYCHOPATHY IN THE TREATMENT
# OF FORENSIC PSYCHIATRIC PATIENTS

ISBN 90 3619 052 5

NUR 740

Cover design: ThTh, Amsterdam


Psychopathy in the treatment of forensic psychiatric patients
Doctoral thesis University of Amsterdam, the Netherlands. — With ref. —
With summary in Dutch.

The research described in this thesis was conducted in the Dr. Henri van der Hoeven Kliniek, center of forensic psychiatry, Utrecht, the Netherlands.

The opinions and statements in this thesis are the responsibility of the author, and such opinions and statements do not necessarily represent the official position of the Dr. Henri van der Hoeven Kliniek.


Key words: psychopathy, PCL-R, forensic psychiatry

# PSYCHOPATHY IN THE TREATMENT OF FORENSIC PSYCHIATRIC PATIENTS

*Assessment, Prevalence, Predictive Validity,*
*and Clinical Implications*

## ACADEMISCH PROEFSCHRIFT

ter verkrijging van de graad van doctor
aan de Universiteit van Amsterdam,
op gezag van de Rector Magnificus
Prof.mr. P.F. van der Heijden
ten overstaan van een door het college van promoties ingestelde
commissie, in het openbaar te verdedigen in de Aula der Universiteit

op vrijdag 8 oktober 2004, te 14.00 uur

door

## MARTIN HILDEBRAND

Geboren te Gouda

**PROMOTORES:**

Mw. Prof.dr. C. de Ruiter

Prof.dr. P.M.G. Emmelkamp

Faculteit der Maatschappij- en Gedragswetenschappen

*This thesis is dedicated
to the memory of the one person who taught me the most
about courage and faith: my little brother, Wilco,*

*and to the memory of my father*

*Power corrupts…*

*Absolute power corrupts absolutely*

(Lord Acton, in a letter to Bishop Mandell Creighton, 1887. "Power tends to corrupt, and absolute power corrupts absolutely. Great men are almost always bad men.")

Het onbegrijpelijke is nou dat als iemand 's iets nieuws van enige *wetenschappelijke* waarde fabriekt, zijn medemensen, vakgenoten voorop, daar afwisselend jaloers en woedend van worden. Ze zullen om strijd roepen dat het product 'niet deugt' of 'zwaar overschat' is. Als hun woede en jaloezie diep genoeg invreten, komen vanzelf de scheldwoorden… de beledigingen… Ze willen dus eigenlijk helemaal niet dat iemand iets bijdraagt aan hun beschaving, waar ze ter meerdere eer en glorie van de eigen status zo hoog van opgeven — tenzij ze de bijdrage zelf verricht hebben… maar dat doen ze nou juist niet…

*Wetenschap* is kennelijk iets om van te profiteren, maar dan moet de bron van het profijt wel anoniem of veilig dood en begraven zijn, want schatplichtigheid aan een levende medebeschaafde, dat is de eigen eer te na.

Vrij naar A.F.Th., *De Movo Tapes* (p. 46) – Em. Querido's uitgeverij, Amsterdam

# CONTENTS

X

# ACKNOWLEDGEMENTS

This thesis has been very much a team effort, and I could not have accomplished it without the talents and dedication of each member of that team. First and foremost, my sincere thanks goes to Corine de Ruiter, Professor of Forensic psychology at the University of Amsterdam. Your generosity, the expertise you shared with me, the autonomy you granted me, and the confidence you showed in me throughout the years, have all been very much appreciated. You genuinely recognize the distinction between complacency and being content, and served as a role model because of your sincere commitment to excellence. Dear Corine, thank you for your unconditional support, understanding, and companionship, having touched my life in a special way and having made me a better person for knowing you.

I thank Paul Emmelkamp, Professor of Clinical psychology at the University of Amsterdam, for agreeing to serve as my second supervisor at a late stage in the process. His suggestions have improved the overall quality of the dissertation. I also would like to extend my appreciation to the committee members Wim Trijsburg, Theo Doreleijers, Robert D. Hare, Ellie Lissenberg, Hjalmar van Marle, Harald Merckelbach, and Aart Schene for reviewing the manuscript. Special recognition needs to go to Dr. Robert D. Hare. His invaluable work provided the inspiration for the subject of this dissertation

My profound gratitude and admiration goes equally to Cécile Vandeputte and Pascalle van der Wolf who have worked with me directly on this research. Dear Cecile, your urban intellect, intriguing observations, and sparkling authenticity have sustained me through easy and tough times. Dear Pascalle, I truly hope that you recognize the important role that your continuing encouraging has played in helping me to achieve my goals. Also, I particularly wish to express my sincere appreciation and gratitude to Vivienne de Vogel for her invaluable help. My grateful thanks also goes to Henk Nijman for his fine collaboration in one of the studies reported here.

While some colleagues have frustrated me in my work, many others have been extremely helpful and invaluable in providing assistance with aspects of the studies reported in this thesis. I particularly wish to acknowledge the contributions of Ellen van den Broek, Ine Kusters, Henriëtte van de Maeden, Marleen Nagtegaal, Lieveken Vester,

Karlijn Vercauteren, Anke Weenink, Baukje van Zaane, Daan van Beek, Martijn Nieuwenhuizen, Pascal Wolters, and Stefan Zwartjes.

This research was carried out in the Dr. Henri van der Hoeven Kliniek in Utrecht, the Netherlands, whose Board of Directors continued to sponsor the study. I want to acknowledge the role of all the patients who participated in the reported studies. I appreciate their willingness to share their personal information; without their efforts, this research could not have been conducted. In addition, the informal discussions with some of them about their experiences in treatment was enlightening.

Next, I want to say thank you to all my new colleagues of the Expertise center for Forensic Psychiatry (EFP) for your confidence and the warm welcome in the past few months.

Thanks are due to my friends, Frieda, Anita, Tanja, Edwin, and Philip, all of whom provided alternative perspectives in times of need. Thank you Leo ("big brother") for lending me *The Da Vinci Code*. Finally, I wish to thank those closest to me who have never wavered in their love and support for me. In particular, my mother, Nel, my two closest friends, Arris and Steven, and Corine.


Life is about dreams, and hope, and courage. The courage to go on, even after those we love have left us. This is not easy. When one is brought low enough repeatedly or for an extended period of time, it becomes increasingly more difficult to imagine oneself happy again or able to push through life with the strength and confidence with which the 'reasonable healthy' go about their daily living. At this point one can teeter on the brink of despair, give up, consider taking one's own life and slide down to the very bottom from which one thinks never to recover. I am deeply grateful to Kees Cornelissen and Jan Scheffer, for invaluable support, enduring patience, thoughtful observations — for helping me to get a life I never would have had otherwise.

# PREFACE

The present thesis comprises several empirical studies with psychopathy, according to the Hare Psychopathy Checklist-Revised (PCL-R; R.D. Hare, 1991), as the central topic.

**Chapter 1** is intended as a general introduction. We touch upon the historical conceptualization of psychopathy as a clinical syndrome; we describe the structure and the psychometric properties of the PCL-R, and we discuss research examining the predictive validity of the PCL-R. Also, the main research questions addressed in this thesis are discussed here, and we describe the setting where the reported research was conducted in some detail.

Next, in **Chapter 2**, we describe a special provision in the Dutch criminal code that allows for a period of treatment (custodial care) following a prison sentence for mentally disordered offenders: *Terbeschikkingstelling* (TBS order).

In **Chapter 3**, a study is presented examining the reliability and factor structure of the Dutch language version of the PCL-R.

The aim of the research presented in **Chapter 4** is to investigate the association between PCL-R psychopathy and mental disorders defined according to the fourth edition of the Diagnostic and Statistical Manual of Mental Disorders (DSM-IV).

In **Chapter 5**, the relationship between PCL-R scores and various types of disruptive behavior during inpatient treatment is investigated.

The main objective of the study presented in **Chapter 6** is to measure treatment progress, by change in indexes of dynamic risk factors.

In **Chapter 7**, the role of the PCL-R and sexual deviance in predicting recidivism in a sample of treated rapists involuntarily admitted between 1975 and 1996, is investigated.

Finally, in **Chapter 8**, the major findings are discussed, a critical analysis of the thesis is presented, recommendations for clinical practice are given, and suggestions for further research on psychopathy are outlined.

The majority of the material presented in the various chapters of this thesis was submitted for publication as separate manuscripts, and therefore some overlap is inevitable. This thesis is based on the following papers:

(1)     De Ruiter, C., & Hildebrand, M. (2003). The dual nature of forensic psychiatric practice: Risk assessment and management under the Dutch TBS-order. In P.J. van Koppen & S.D. Penrod (Eds.), *Adversarial versus inquisitorial justice: Psychological perspectives on criminal justice systems* (pp. 91-106). New York: Kluwer/Plenum. (Chapter 2)

(2)     Hildebrand, M., de Ruiter, C., de Vogel, V., & van der Wolf, P. (2002). Reliability and factor structure of the Dutch language version of Hare's Psychopathy Checklist-Revised. *International Journal of Forensic Mental Health*, *1*, 139-154. (Chapter 3)

(3)     Hildebrand, M., & de Ruiter, C. (2004). PCL-R psychopathy and its relation to DSM-IV Axis I and Axis II disorders in a sample of male forensic psychiatric patients in the Netherlands. *International Journal of Law and Psychiatry*, *27*, 233-248. (Chapter 4)

(4)     Hildebrand, M., de Ruiter, C., & Nijman, H. (2004). PCL-R psychopathy predicts disruptive behavior among male offenders in a Dutch forensic psychiatric hospital. *Journal of Interpersonal Violence*, *19*, 13-29. (Chapter 5)

(5)     Hildebrand, M., de Ruiter, C., & van Zaane, B. *Psychopathy and change in dynamic risk factors during inpatient treatment.* Submitted for publication. (Chapter 6)

(6)     Hildebrand, M., de Ruiter, C., & de Vogel, V. (2004). Psychopathy and sexual deviance in treated rapists: Association with sexual and non-sexual recidivism. *Sexual Abuse: A Journal of Research and Treatment*, *16*, 1-24. (Chapter 7)

The papers were pre-printed or printed with kind permission from Kluwer Academic/Plenum Publishers, Elsevier Science Ltd, Sage Publications, Inc., and the International Association of Forensic Mental Health Services.

CHAPTER 1

THE CONSTRUCT OF PSYCHOPATHY

## SUMMARY

Chapter 1 offers an introduction to the following chapters. After the historical conceptualization of psychopathy as a clinical syndrome is touched upon, we describe the development, structure, administration and scoring of the PCL-R, as well as its psychometric properties. We review research examining the validity of the PCL-R in terms of covariation with other psychological measures and physiological processes, and we turn our focus on the utility of the PCL-R in the prediction of institutional misbehavior, treatment outcome, and criminal recidivism. It is concluded that (PCL-R) psychopathy is an important factor in understanding and predicting criminal conduct. Specifically, (PCL-R) psychopathy is associated with increased risk of violent and aggressive behavior, disruptive behavior, high rates of (different types of) recidivism, and poor treatment outcome.

Next, the main research questions addressed in this thesis are outlined, and the setting where the research was conducted, the Dr. Henri van der Hoeven Kliniek in Utrecht, the Netherlands, is described in some detail — with special reference to psychological assessment procedures used to periodically evaluate treatment progress.

# INTRODUCTION

Both the nature and the breadth of the defining features of psychopathic personality disorder have generated considerable confusion among both researchers and clinicians (e.g., Blackburn, 1988; Hare, Hart, & Harpur, 1991; Holmes, 1992; Millon, Simonsen, & Birketh-Smith, 1998). During the past 200 years, scholars have formulated and reformulated the construct of psychopathy innumerable times (e.g., Cleckley, 1941/1982; Hare, 1991, 1993; Millon et al., 1998). Amidst all of these formulations, some researchers have asserted that the disorder is "a myth...a nonexistent entity" (Karpman, 1948, p. 523) or "a mythical entity" Blackburn (1988, p. 511), whereas others argued that, at the very least, the construct of psychopathy cannot be regarded as a useful construct either from a clinical or from a theoretical perspective (Gunn, 1998). Given the compelling (mainly North American) evidence regarding both the clinical value of the construct and its theoretical coherence, Hare (1998a) states that "these views typically have an armchair quality about them, and are held with surprising certitude and tenacity" (p. 188).

It is true that the etiology, dynamics, and conceptual boundaries of the disorder are the subject of debate, but at the same time there is a consistent clinical tradition concerning its core affective, interpersonal, and behavioral attributes, which cuts across a broad spectrum of professionals, including psychiatrists, correction workers, psychologists, and experimental psychopathologists (e.g., Blair, 1995, 2001; Blair, Jones, Clark, & Smith, 1997; Blair et al., 2002; Cleckley, 1941/1982; Flor, Birbaumer, Hermann, Ziegler, & Patrick, 2002; Hare, 1993, 1996, 1998b; Hart, 1998; Kiehl et al., 2001; Lilienfeld, 1994; Livesley, 1998; McCord & McCord, 1964; Meloy, 1988; Millon, 1969; Raine, 2001; Raine, Lencz, Bihrle, LaCasse, & Colletti, 2000; Schmitt & Newman, 1999; Tennent, Tennent, Prins, & Bedford, 1990). Nevertheless, until recently, the lack of psychometrically sound procedures for diagnosing the disorder has hindered the development of a body of replicable, theoretically meaningful research findings, as well as the acceptance of psychopathy as an important clinical construct with practical implications.

## HISTORICAL CONCEPTUALIZATION OF PSYCHOPATHY
## AS A CLINICAL SYNDROME[1]

More than 200 years ago, Phillipe Pinel (1801/1962), a French physician and pioneer in the field of mental disorders, encountered unusual cases not fitting any contemporary classification for mental disturbance. Characterized by relatively normal intellectual functions — imagination, judgment, memory, perception — but a pronounced disorder of affect, blind impulse to acts of violence, even murderous fury, he described the syndrome as *manie sans délire* (Pinel, 1801/1962). Other clinicians noted similar cases of "moral insanity" (Prichard, 1835), in whom clear thought coexisted with affective disturbance and socially deviant behaviors (Rush, 1812).

Typologies for classifying criminal behavior in general and psychopathy in particular were as numerous as the terms (e.g., Partridge, 1930). They often reflected individual moral beliefs or the psychological *Zeitgeist* of the period. In 1891, the German psychiatrist Koch proposed the term "constitutional psychopathic inferiority" as a more acceptable alternative to Pritchards' (1935) term "moral insanity". Koch asserted that the term "psychopathic" was more appropriate because it more accurately conveyed his belief that the disorder was a psychological abnormality with a physiological basis that did not amount to insanity (Blackburn, 1988; Millon et al., 1998).

Early on, clinicians believed degenerative processes underlied most mental disturbances (e.g., *dementia praecox*). Influenced by this bias, those who described psychopathy ignored information concerning personality (e.g., Lewis, 1974; Maudsley, 1874). Psychopathy became a wastebasket category for all personality deviations. The poorly defined category produced a plethora of descriptive terms — e.g., constitutional inferiority, constitutional psychopathic inferiority, constitutional psychopathic personality, psychopathy, constitutional defectiveness, neurotic constitution, sociopathy (Partridge, 1930) — which indicated the lack of a clearly defined syndrome. The social context for defining psychopathy was embedded within a 19th-century concern to treat the mentally ill

---

[1] For extensive reviews on the concepts and theories of psychopathic personality disorder, see, for example, Millon, Simonsen, & Birket-Smith (1998).

offender separate from the non-mentally ill criminal. The distinction between the 'mad' and the 'bad' continues to be a struggle for many forensic clinicians today.

Although neurobiological roots were still hypothesized, Kraepelin's (1915) adoption of the term "psychopathic personality" led to a decline in the use of terms that suggested a degenerative process (Gacono, 1988). In 1909, Birnbaum, a German researcher, suggested that the term "sociopath" might be a more accurate label for most of these individuals (Millon et al., 1998). Birnbaum hypothesized that antisocial behavior was rarely the result of intrinsic personality traits and/or characteristics, but generally reflected the operation of societal forces on the individual (Millon et al., 1998). In the United States, the term "sociopath" was first introduced by Partridge. In 1930, Partridge hypothesized that psychopathy was characterized exclusively by social maladjustment. Therefore, he asserted that the term "sociopath" would be a more accurate and applicable label to describe these individuals. D.K. Henderson (1939) agreed with Patridge's basic conclusions regarding the nature of psychopathy (Millon et al., 1998). However, he asserted that psychopathy should be divided into three clinical subtypes: (1) the predominantly aggressive; (2) the predominantly passive or inadequate, and (3) the predominantly creative (Millon et al., 1998). One of D.K. Henderson's unique contributions to the conceptualization of psychopathy was his assertion that not all psychopaths were criminals (Millon et al., 1998), a notion later expanded by Cleckley (1941/1982).

Eleven years after Partridge's (1930) review article in which he identified the confusion surrounding the term psychopathy, a seminal book on the psychopathic personality was published by Cleckley (1941), *The mask of sanity*. To summarize what he thought to be the essential features of *primary* psychopaths (see below), Cleckley formulated a list of 16 core characteristics of psychopathy that still is widely accepted today as the best definition of the psychopath (Table 1).

TABLE 1
*Cleckley's 16 Criteria for Psychopathy*

---

**Key features**

Unresponsiveness in general interpersonal relations
Superficial charm and good intelligence
Absence of delusions and other signs of irrational thinking
Absence of "nervousness" or other neurotic manifestations
Lack of remorse and shame
Poor judgment and failure to learn from experience
Pathological egocentricity and incapacity for love
General poverty in major affective reactions
Inadequately motivated antisocial behavior

**Other characteristics**

Impersonal, trivial, and poorly integrated sex life
Unreliability
Failure to follow any life plan
Untruthfulness and insincerity
Suicide rarely carried out
Specific loss of insight
Fantastic and uninviting behavior with drink and sometimes without

---

*Source.* From Cleckley (1982, p. 204). We used the wording of "Key features" and "Other characteristics" from Andrews and Bonta (2003). *The psychology of criminal conduct* (3rd ed). Cincinnati, OH: Anderson.

Cleckley expanded on early organic and behavioral conceptualizations of psychopathy (Gacono, 1988). Although postulating a constitutional deficit, Cleckley's trait descriptions provided clinical criteria without links to a degenerative disorder. He believed the psychopath suffered a semantic problem in that he was unable to process or internalize the affective components of human interaction (Cleckley, 1941/1982). Or, as Johns & Quay (1962) cogently stated, "the psychopath can thus be said to be one who knows the words but not the music; the denotative meaning of words and phrase may be intact but the connotative emotional or motivational component is lost" (p. 217).

Cleckley argued that moral feelings and compunctions must be learned and that this learning process is guided and enforced by the power of emotional feelings. When these normal feelings are attenuated, the development of morality — the very mechanism of socialization — is compromised.

McCord and McCord (1964) stated that the defining characteristics of psychopathic individuals are "guiltlessness and lovelessness", and they cautioned that an individual should not be categorized as a psychopath unless the individual demonstrates these two essential symptoms in various aspects of functioning, while according to Hare (1970),

> Most clinical descriptions of the psychopath make some sort of reference to his egocentricity, lack of empathy, and inability to form warm, emotional relationships with others characteristics that lead him to treat others as objects instead of as persons and prevent him from experiencing guilt and remorse for having done so. (p. 14)

Millon (1969, 1975) attempted to anchor psychopathic behavior to learning and psychological dynamics (see Millon et al., 1998). He described psychopaths as being "self-assertive, temperamentally hostile, socially forceful, and intimidating" (Millon et al., 1998, p. 23). In his view, deficiency in concern for other people is the essential clinical symptom of psychopathy, which is essentially a combination of narcissism and antisocial behavior. According to Millon, a passive variant of the psychopathic individual's lack of concern for others is evident in the self-focus of the narcissistic personality, while an active variant of the psychopath's lack of concern for others is evident in the destructive behavior of the antisocial personality.

Research with psychopaths, which started in the mid 1940s, suggested the existence of two distinct types of psychopathy: *primary* and *secondary* psychopathy (Karpman, 1946, 1948; see also Blackburn, 1975; Doren, 1987; Eysenck, 1964; Karpman, 1941, 1961).[2] Karpman (1946) defined primary psychopaths primarily in terms of personality characteristics and secondary psychopaths primarily in terms of emotional disturbances and resulting impulsivity. He argued that the primary psychopath's characteristics are so deeply ingrained that the only reasonable explanation is that the individual was born as a psychopath. Secondary psychopaths, on the other hand, do experience guilt and are able to

---

[2] For the sake of completeness, we mention here that there have been numerous attempts to classify criminal offenders and/or psychopaths into subtypes (For an extensive review, see Megargee & Bohn, 1979). According to Lykken (1995), typologies have usually been based on factors as the instant offense, criminal career pattern, social class, and on the basis of psychoanalytic or developmental theories (e.g., Millon & Davis, 1998). However, more empirical typologies have also been developed (e.g., Blackburn, 1975, 1986; Megargee & Bohn, 1979; Quay, 1977).

form attachments. According to Karpman (1948), secondary psychopaths engage in antisocial behavior because of underlying emotional disorder that is typically manifested as extreme impulsivity. Other researchers have referred to secondary psychopaths as "symptomatic" or "neurotic" psychopaths (e.g., Doren, 1987). According to Levenson, Kiehl, and Fitzpatrick (1995), secondary psychopaths are more likely to come into contact with the criminal justice (or forensic mental health) system because of their characteristic emotional disorders and impulsivity. The debate about the distinction between primary and secondary is of importance because it touches upon the notion of the treatability of psychopaths. Those with a capacity for emotionality and with some conscience may be more amenable to treatment (Blackburn, 1993; Eysenck, 1998) and less likely to act violently (Herpertz & Sass, 2000).

The assertion of Levenson et al. (1995) regarding the subtypes of psychopathy and the likelihood of engaging in antisocial behavior relates to Cleckley's clinical observation that criminal behavior was not an essential characteristic of psychopathy. Others since Cleckley also believed that 'not all psychopaths ended up in prison' (Babiak, 1995, 2000; Bursten, 1972, 1973; Millon, 1981). According to Andrews and Bonta (2003), accepting the assumption that a psychopath is not necessarily a criminal, holds that "an etiological explanation of crime may not serve as an explanation of psychopathy, and vice versa, and assessment and treatment methods for psychopaths and criminals should be substantially different" (p. 370).

Finally, Weiner (1991) hypothesized, with some empirical support, that many 'noncriminal' psychopaths manifest similar superego deficits as criminal psychopaths, but maintain more intact ego functions, such as impulse control. This is consistent with observations that these individuals may not meet the behavioral criteria for antisocial personality disorder (ASPD) but do often meet the threshold criteria for other personality disorders (i.e., paranoid or narcissistic personality disorder) (Wulach, 1988). Currently, however, our knowledge base regarding the behavioral, interpersonal, and affective characteristics of noninstitutionalized psychopaths is significantly limited.

## DSM CRITERIA

As is evident from the foregoing discussion, the construct of psychopathy has been conceptualized in various ways throughout the past 200 years. The changing conceptualization of psychopathy is reflected quite clearly in the nosological terminology and diagnostic criteria sets contained in the various editions of the *Diagnostic and Statistical Manual of Mental Disorders* (DSM; American Psychiatric Association [APA], 1952, 1968, 1980, 1987, 1994). In the first *DSM*, the term personality disorder was used for the most general classification of personality disturbance, of which four subtypes were identified: *personality pattern disturbances*, *personality trait disturbances*, *sociopathic personality disturbances*, and *special symptom reactions*. Sociopathic personality disturbances described a variety of conditions, such as sexual deviation, alcoholism, and 'antisocial" and 'dissocial' reactions. The 'antisocial reaction' diagnosis was given to those individuals

> [...] who are always in trouble, profiting neither from experience nor punishment and maintaining no loyalties to any person, group or code. They are frequently callous and hedonistic, showing marked emotional immaturity with lack of sense of responsibility, lack of judgment, and an ability to rationalize their behavior so that it appears warranted, reasonable, and justified. (APA, 1952, p. 38)

The antisocial diagnosis closely resembled the classic psychopath (Jenkins, 1960). The reactive aspect of the diagnosis, however, suggested a fundamentally learned response to the slings and arrows of the environment — the original premise of Birnbaum (1914) who coined the term sociopath.

The *DSM-II* (APA, 1968) eliminated the reactivity criteria, presented a number of personality disorders, and subsumed antisocial and dissocial reactions under the rubric of "antisocial personality". ASPD was distinguished by unsocialized and antisocial behavior. Incapable of significant loyalty to individual, group, or social values they were described as callous, irresponsible, selfish, impulsive, unable to feel guilt or to learn from experience and punishment. They demonstrated poor frustration tolerance and blamed others, while offering plausible rationalizations for their behavior (APA, 1968). These changes in *DSM-*

*II* were based on the groundbreaking empirical research on delinquents of Lee Robins (1966). Her work provided a social deviancy model of antisocial personality, in contrast to Cleckley's "personality" or trait model.

Although the *DSM-II* maintained some traits incorporated in more traditional descriptions of psychopathy (e.g., Hare et al., 1991; Karpman, 1961; Millon, 1981), the fixed set of behavioral criteria in the *DSM-III* (APA, 1980) firmly endorsed a social deviance model (L. Robins, 1966) and eschewed most trait descriptions. A definition of ASPD was created that consisted largely of determining whether the subject had participated in a number of criminal or antisocial acts in childhood and in adulthood (APA, 1980). The *DSM-III* and *DSM-III-R* (APA, 1987) criteria did not explicitly include traits such as selfishness, egocentricity, callousness, manipulativeness, and lack of empathy. These characteristics were found in the criteria for narcissistic personality disorder. The revision of the third edition emphasized an early onset (< 15 years) of continuous and chronic antisocial behavior that persisted into adult life, while eliminating reference to specific traits. Thus, *DSM-III* and *DSM-III-R* moved further away from the psychopathic traits that had been described by Cleckley.[3]

In the most recent edition of the DSM, *DSM-IV* (APA, 1994), criteria for ASPD, although simplified (seven items), again firmly endorsed the social deviance model. Table 2 lists the criteria for the *DSM-IV* ASPD, and the criteria for dissocial personality disorder as defined in the 10th edition of the *International Classification of Diseases* (ICD-10; World Health Organization [WHO], 1992).

---

[3] Psychopathy has also been compared with a diagnosis of dissocial personality disorder as defined in the 10th edition of the *International Classification of Diseases* (ICD-10; World Health Organization [WHO], 1990).

**TABLE 2**

*Criteria for DSM-IV Antisocial and ICD-10 Dissocial Personality Disorder*

| DSM-IV | ICD-10 |
|---|---|
| A. Antisocial behavior since age 15, as indicated by three or more of the following:<br><br>1. Repeated criminal acts<br>2. Deceitfulness<br>3. Impulsivity<br>4. Irritability and aggressiveness<br>5. Recklessness<br>6. Irresponsibility<br>7. Lack of remorse<br><br>B. Current age at least 18 years<br><br>C. Conduct disorder before age 15, indicated by clinically significant impairment in social, academic or occupational functioning resulting from three or more of the following:<br><br>1. Bullied<br>2. Fought<br>3. Used weapons<br>4. Cruel to people<br>5. Cruel to animals<br>6. Robbed<br>7. Forced sex on others<br>8. Set fires<br>9. Destroyed property<br>10. Broke and entered<br>11. Lied<br>12. Stole<br>13. Stayed out late<br>14. Ran away from home<br>15. Truant | A. Callous unconcern for the feelings of others and lack of the capacity for empathy<br><br>B. Gross and persistent attitude of irresponsibility and disregard for social norms, rules, and obligations<br><br>C. Incapacity to maintain enduring relationships<br><br>D. Very low tolerance to frustration and a low threshold for discharge of aggression, including violence<br><br>E. Incapacity to experience guilt and to profit from experience, particularly punishment<br><br>F. Marked proneness to blame others or to offer plausible rationalizations for the behavior bringing the subject into conflict with society<br><br>G. Persistent irritability |

D. Occurrence of antisocial behavior not exclusively during the course of schizophrenia or manic episodes

*Source.* Adapted from American Psychiatric Association (1994). *Diagnostic and Statistical Manual of Mental Disorders* (4th ed.). Washington, DC: Author; World Health Organization (1992). *International Classification of Diseases* (10th ed.). Geneva, Switzerland: Author.

ASPD is defined as an obdurate penchant for engaging in negativistic and destructive conduct starting early in life and continuing in adulthood (*DSM-IV*, p. 645). In order to qualify for the diagnosis, a person has to show a persistent pattern of misconduct — that is, early evidence of conduct disorder. Another prerequisite is that the misconduct did not occur during the course of schizophrenia or manic episodes. The *DSM-IV* text says that the pervasive pattern of disregard for, and violation of, the rights of others "has also been referred to as psychopathy, sociopathy or dissocial personality disorder" (p. 645). Indeed, the text makes many references to the personality traits traditionally associated with psychopathy:

> Individuals with antisocial personality disorder frequently lack empathy and tend to be callous, cynical, and contemptuous of the feelings, rights, and sufferings of others. They may have an inflated and arrogant self-appraisal (...) and may be excessively opinionated, self-assured, or cocky. They may display a glib, superficial charm and can be quite voluble and verbally facile. Lack of empathy, inflated self-appraisal, and superficial charm are features that have been commonly included in traditional conceptions of psychopathy and may be particularly distinguishing of antisocial personality disorder in prison or forensic settings where criminal, delinquent, or aggressive acts are likely to be nonspecific. These individuals may also be irresponsible and exploitative in their sexual relationships. They may have a history of many sexual partners and may never have sustained a monogamous relationship. (p. 647)

The change in focus in the diagnostic criteria contained in the different editions of the DSM not only reflects the evolving conceptualization of psychopathy, but it also reflects the divergent approaches that researchers have taken in the investigation of psychopathy (Lilienfeld, 1994; Reise & Oliver, 1994). Specifically, while some researchers have focused primarily on personality traits in defining psychopathy (e.g., Cleckley, 1941/1982; Jenkins, 1960), others have focused primarily on behavioral characteristics in defining psychopathy (e.g., Karpman, 1961), and still others have emphasized both personality traits and behavioral characteristics in defining psychopathy (e.g., Hare, 1980, 1985).

The advocates of the personality-based approach to defining psychopathy believe that psychopathy should be viewed primarily as a constellation of personality traits

(Lilienfeld, 1994). They argue that this has two important advantages (Reise & Oliver, 1994). First, individuals defined as psychopaths according to the personality-based approach are psychologically homogenous (Reise & Oliver, 1994). Second, the personality-based approach is better able to identify the 'successful' psychopaths who have not come into contact with the mental health or criminal justice systems (Reise & Oliver, 1994).

The advocates of the behavior-based approach to psychopathy believe that psychopathy should be defined primarily with reference to a history of agreed-upon antisocial behaviors (Lilienfeld, 1994), and is reflected in the diagnostic criteria sets contained in the three most recent editions of the DSM (APA, 1980, 1987, 1994). Advocates of the behavior-based approach to defining psychopathy argue that it has two major advantages over the personality-based approach (Reise & Oliver, 1994). First, the behavior-based approach does not require many psychological inferences on the part of the clinician. Second, the behavior-based approach results in high diagnostic interrater reliability (Reise & Oliver, 1994).

Finally, some researchers have emphasized both personality traits and behavioral characteristics. The advocates of this approach believe that psychopathy is most appropriately viewed as a combination of personality traits and behavioral characteristics (Lilienfeld, 1994).

## THE HARE PSYCHOPATHY CHECKLIST-REVISED (PCL-R)

At a conceptual or linguistic level, psychopathic personality disorder is synonymous with antisocial, dissocial and sociopathic personality disorder; they are simply different terms for the same disorder. This is explicitly recognized in the *DSM-IV* (APA, 1994, p. 645). At an *operational* level, however, it must be emphasized that the various diagnostic criteria sets for antisocial, dissocial, sociopathic, and psychopathic personality disorder are *not* equivalent.

An adequate diagnosis of psychopathy must be based on the full range of relevant symptomatology. An exclusive focus on behavioral symptoms (i.e., irresponsibility, delinquency), for example, to the exclusion of affective and interpersonal symptoms may lead to overdiagnosing of psychopathy in criminal populations and underdiagnosing in non-criminals (Hare et al., 1991; Lilienfeld, 1994; Widiger & Corbitt, 1995). To ensure accurate diagnosis, psychopathy should be assessed using expert observer (i.e., clinical) ratings, based on a review of case history materials —such as criminal and psychological/ psychiatric records— and supplemented with interviews or behavioral observations whenever possible (Hare, 1991). The next section briefly addresses the development, structure, administration, and scoring of the PCL-R.

## PCL-R: DEVELOPMENT, STRUCTURE, ADMINISTRATION, AND SCORING

*Development.* In the late 1970s, expanding on Cleckley's conceptualization of psychopathy, and adding items related to antisocial behavior, Hare and his colleagues began developing a research tool for operationalizing the construct psychopathy — the 22-item Psychopathy Checklist (PCL; Hare, 1980). According to Hare, the "impetus for the development of the PCL was the recognition that traditional assessment procedures, including those based on clinical diagnosis and on self-report inventories, lacked demonstrated reliability and validity" (Hare, 1991, p.1). Research with the PCL demonstrated that it was a reliable assessment measure with strong psychometric properties, and it was rapidly adopted by numerous researchers and clinicians as the gold standard in psychopathy assessment measures (e.g., Hare, 1991; Hare & McPherson, 1984; Hart, Hare, & Harpur, 1992; Schroeder, Schroeder, & Hare, 1993). The PCL was revised in 1985 and formally published in 1991 as the 20-item Hare PCL-R (Hare, 1991), and has been initially validated with data from North American samples of prison inmates and forensic psychiatric patients (see reviews by Fulero, 1995; Stone, 1995). Currently, the PCL-R is regarded as the most widely-accepted and empirically-validated instrument for measuring psychopathy in both correctional and forensic psychiatric populations (Hare, 1991; Rice, 1997).

*Structure.* At least initially, PCL-R items were considered to be underpinned by two distinct but correlated factors (e.g., Hare, 1991; Hare et al., 1990; Harpur, Hare, & Hakstian, 1989; Harpur, Hakstian, & Hare, 1988; Hart et al., 1992). The first factor (8 items) reflects the interpersonal and affective features of psychopathy, and has been labeled "Selfish, callous and remorseless use of others" (Hare, 1991; Hare et al., 1990).

Factor 1 is closely related to the core personality features of psychopathy as articulated by Cleckley (1941/1982), as well as to *DSM-IV* narcissistic personality disorder (Harpur et al., 1988; Hart, Forth, & Hare, 1991). Factor 2 (nine items) primarily measures the (antisocial) behavioral aspects of psychopathy and has been labeled "Chronically unstable and antisocial lifestyle." Factor 2 is closely associated with a *DSM-IV* diagnosis of ASPD (e.g., Harpur et al., 1988).[4] The remaining three items of the PCL-R (promiscuous sexual behavior, many short-term marital relationships and criminal versatility) did not load on either factor (Hare, 1991; Hare et al., 1990). Table 3 presents the 20 items of the PCL-R and their location in the traditional two-factor structure.

**TABLE 3**
*Items in the Hare Psychopathy Checklist-Revised (PCL-R; Hare, 1991) and Their Location in the Traditional Two-Factor Structure*

| Factor 1 | Factor 2 | Additional items |
|---|---|---|
| 1. Glibness / superficial charm | 3. Need for stimulation / proneness to boredom | 11. Promiscuous sexual behavior |
| 2. Grandiose sense of self-worth | 9. Parasitic lifestyle | 17. Many short-term marital relationship |
| 4. Pathological lying | 10. Poor behavioral controls | 20. Criminal versatility |
| 5. Conning or manipulative | 12. Early behavioral problems | |
| 6. Lack of remorse or guilt | 13. Lack of realistic, long-term goals | |
| 7. Shallow affect | 14. Impulsivity | |
| 8. Callous / lack of empathy | 15. Irresponsibility | |
| 16. Failure to accept responsibility for own actions | 18. Juvenile delinquency | |
| | 19. Revocation of conditional release | |

*Note.* Additional items = items that do not load on either factor.
*Source.* Adapted from Hare, R.D. (1991). *The Hare Psychopathy Checklist-Revised.* Toronto, Canada: Multi-Health Systems.

Recent re-analysis, by means of Item Response Theory (IRT) and confirmatory factor analyses (CFA), suggests that a *three*-factor model that only uses the 13 items of the PCL-R that deal with personality traits (rather than delinquency and social deviance) might actually provide a better fit than the traditional two-factor model (Cooke & Michie, 2001).

---

[4] Recently, the Hare Psychopathy Checklist-Revised (PCL-R™): 2nd edition is published.

In essence, the three-factor model of Cooke and Michie (2001) posits, that a coherent superordinate factor (i.e., psychopathy), is underpinned by an interpersonal (*Deceitful interpersonal style*), affective (*Deficient affective experience*), and behavioral (*Impulsive and irresponsible behavioral style*) factor. In a series of seven studies, this three-factor model of psychopathy was developed and cross-validated in North American ($n$ = 2067) and Scottish ($n$ = 596) forensic and correctional subsamples using the PCL-R and then crossvalidated on alternative measures of psychopathy, including the 12-item Psychopathy Checklist: Screening Version (PCL:SV; Hart, Cox, & Hare, 1995), and the psychopathy criteria from the *DSM-IV* field trial. In each study, the fit of the proposed three-factor model was compared with that of several competing models, including the original two-factor model. The three-factor model was found to fit the data consistently and to fit significantly better than competing models. Table 4 presents the three-factor hierarchical model of Cooke and Michie (2001).

TABLE 4
*Cooke and Michie's (2001) Three-Factor Model Derived from the PCL-R*

| Factor 1 (Arrogant and Deceitful Interpersonal Style) | Factor 2 (Deficient Emotional Experience) | Factor 3 (Impulsive and Irresponsible Behavioral Style) |
|---|---|---|
| 1. Glibness / superficial charm<br>2. Grandiose sense of self-worth<br>4. Pathological lying<br>5. Conning / manipulative | 6. Lack of remorse or guilt<br>7. Shallow affect<br>8. Callous / lack of empathy<br>16. Failure to accept responsibility for own actions | 3. Need for stimulation / proneness to boredom<br>9. Parasitic lifestyle<br>13. Lack of realistic, long-term goals<br>14. Impulsivity<br>15. Irresponsibility |

*Note.* PCL-R = Psychopathy Checklist-Revised.

The most important difference between the Hare PCL-R and DSM-IV's ASPD is on the emotional-interpersonal dimension (Hare, 1998a).[5] The diagnostic criteria for ASPD

---

[5] The differences between these two diagnostic traditions are discussed extensively elsewhere (e.g., Cunningham & Reidy, 1998; Hare et al., 1991; Hart & Hare, 1997; Lilienfeld, 1994; Lilienfeld, Purcell, & Jones-Alexander, 1997; Widiger & Corbitt, 1995).

tend to focus more narrowly on overt delinquent behavior (e.g., APA, 1980, 1987, 1994. In contrast, diagnostic criteria for psychopathy typically include a broad range of affective, behavioral, and interpersonal characteristics (e.g., Cleckley, 1941/1982; Hare, 1970, 1980, 1991; Hart et al., 1995). Cooke and Michie (1997, 1999; also Cooke, Michie, Hart, & Hare, 1999) concluded that the interpersonal and affective items of the PCL-R are of greater importance than the behavioral characteristics for taxon identification or behavioral prediction. Recently, however, Skilling, Harris, Rice, & Quinsey (2002) reported that, when scored as continuous measures, the association between PCL-R and *DSM-IV* criteria of ASPD is extremely high, which means that "persistently antisocial individuals not only exhibit such [...] characteristics as antisocial behavior beginning early in life, but (with extremely high likelihood) also exhibit psychopathic glibness, superficiality, failure to take responsibility, shallow affect, and so on" (p. 35).

At the heart of the diagnostic controversy between psychopathy and ASPD has been the question of whether the latent constellation of traits proposed by each group represented taxonic (i.e., categories) or nontaxonic (i.e., dimensions, factors) phenotypic indicators (Meehl, 1995). Indeed, the question whether psychopaths are qualitatively different from nonpsychopathic criminals or whether all criminals are psychopaths to a certain extent is important. Is psychopathy a discrete personality construct (a taxon) or a continuous dimension of personality? Harris, Rice, and Quinsey (1994) concluded that the taxonic characteristics were empirically documented by the PCL-R. Specifically, Factor 2 items and other childhood variables were found to be associated with a taxon underlying psychopathy. These findings are inconsistent with those of Cooke and Michie (1997) who concluded that Factor 1 of the PCL-R was the most sensitive discriminator of psychopathy. Harris et al. (1994) determined that PCL-R scores of 19-20 optimally maximized the number of false positives and false negatives. Harris, Rice, and Cormier (1991) suggested a PCL-R cutoff of 25 optimally categorized a taxon for psychopathy and criminal recidivism. However, Harris et al. (1994) recommended that different cutoff scores be used for different forensic questions. For research purposes, however, a score of 30 is generally recommended as indicative of psychopathy (Hare, 1991), although researchers have used scores varying from 15 (Seto & Barbaree, 1999) to 32 (Serin, Peters, & Barbaree, 1990). Meloy and Gacono (1995) even recommended a cutting score of 33 for clinical purposes, taking the standard error of the instrument, i.e. 3 points, into account. The variability reported in various studies has left the controversy insufficiently examined.

*Administration and scoring.* The PCL-R is completed on the basis of a semi-structured interview and collateral (file) information.[6] The interview is conducted for two reasons. First, the interview is conducted to obtain specific historical information across several domains of functioning that is necessary to score some PCL-R items (Hare, 1991). The interview covers several areas of the individual's functioning, such as school adjustment, work history, future goals, finances, family background, sexual and intimate relationships, child and adolescent antisocial behavior and adult delinquency. Second, the interview provides the examiner with an opportunity to observe the individual's interpersonal style and behavioral characteristics over a reasonably long period of time (Hare, 1991). The review of collateral information serves to (1) enable the examiner to evaluate the credibility of the information provided by the individual during the interview; (2) it assists the examiner in determining whether the interpersonal style displayed by the subject during the interview is representative of the subject's usual behavior, and (3) it provides the examiner with the primary data for scoring several of the PCR-R items (e.g., criminal versatility, juvenile delinquency).

Each of the PCL-R items is scored on a 3-point ordinal scale (0 = *item does not apply*, 1 = *item applies to a certain extent*, 2 = *item definitely applies*), according to the scoring criteria contained in the PCL-R administration and scoring manual (Hare, 1991). Examiners should score each of the 20 PCL-R items on the basis of the individual's lifetime functioning. Hare (1991) warns that the PCL-R items should not be scored solely on the basis of the individual's functioning at the time of the evaluation. If there is insufficient information to score a particular item, the item can be omitted. According to the PCL-R manual, up to five items can be omitted without invalidating the PCL-R total score. Up to two items can be omitted on each PCL-R Factor without invalidating the respective Factor scores. The total score can range from 0 to 40, reflecting the degree to which an individual resembles the prototypical psychopath. Hare (1991) suggested a cutoff

---

[6] Considerable research with the PCL-R suggests that accurate PCL-R ratings may be based solely on file information, that is, if there is sufficient high-quality information (Grann, Långström, Tengström, & Stålenheim, 1998; Hare, 1991; Koivisto & Haapasalo, 1996; Wong, 1988; see also Chapter 7).

score of 30 or more to assign a clinical diagnosis of psychopathy. In European research, however, a cutoff score of 26 is often used.[7]

## CLINICAL UTILITY OF THE PCL-R

According to Cooke (1998), the validity of a clinical construct has to be evaluated in relation to a wide range of criteria (e.g., Blashfield & Draguns, 1976; Kendell, 1989; E. Robins & Guze, 1970), including: (1) psychometric properties; (2) evidence of covariation between the construct and abnormalities of a psychological, physiological, or biochemical nature, and (3) predictive validity in terms of treatment outcome and/or future behavior. Below, we will briefly review how well the PCL-R performs against these criteria.

### PSYCHOMETRIC PROPERTIES

There is compelling evidence that Hare's construct of psychopathy has substantial validity. Psychometric analyses based on classical test theory and item response theory (IRT) indicate that the PCL-R has excellent psychometric properties (Hare et al., 1990; Cooke & Michie, 1997, 2001). It is found that PCL-R psychopathy can be diagnosed as reliably as most (acute) mental disorders (and more reliably than other personality disorders) in clinical and research settings (e.g., Hare, 1991; Widiger et al., 1996). Of the studies providing reliability statistics in the meta-analysis of Hemphill, Hare, and Wong (1998), interrater or intraclass correlation coefficients all exceeded .80. Both factor analytic studies and IRT modeling have demonstrated that the diverse manifestations of the disorder — the affective, interpersonal, and behavioral characteristics — are underpinned by coherent latent traits (Hare et al., 1990; Cooke, 1995; Cooke, Kosson, & Michie, 2001; Cooke & Michie, 1997, 2001; Cooke et al., 1999). There is no evidence that the construct validity of psychopathy is unduly affected by race or culture (e.g., Cooke, 1995, 1996; Cooke et al., 2001; Kosson, Smith, & Newman, 1990).

---

[7] Therefore, in our studies (Chapters 3-7), we also used a cutoff of 26 to assign a clinical diagnosis of psychopathy.

**COVARIATION WITH MEASURES OF PSYCHOLOGICAL AND PHYSIOLOGICAL PROCESSES**

There is also convincing evidence for the validity of the psychopathy construct in terms of covariation with psychological measures and physiological processes.[8] Several lines of research are of particular importance. First, although no evidence has been found that (PCL-R) psychopaths suffer from gross cerebral impairment (e.g., Smith, Arnett, & Newman, 1992), they show impaired performance on cognitive tasks related to passive-avoidance learning (e.g., Howland, Kosson, Patterson, & Newman, 1993; Lapierre, Braun, & Hodgins, 1995; Newman, Kosson, & Patterson, 1992). Hare and Craigen (1974) found that psychopaths exhibit unusual patterns of physiological arousal, particularly in anticipation of noxious stimuli (see also, among others, Arnett, Howland, Smith, & Newman, 1993; Raine & Venables, 1988a, 1988b). They display anticipatory heart rate acceleration while awaiting an inevitable, aversive stimulus, but they do not display any significant increase in electrodermal response. Hare (1978) interpreted this pattern of anticipatory physiological arousal as evidence of an adaptive coping response that helps psychopaths to ignore selectively cues of impending punishment but that also makes them susceptible to overfocusing on reward cues. Deficient conditioning leads to an inability to learn from punishment experiences and to develop avoidance learning (Herpertz & Sass, 2000).

Also, research with a variety of paradigms (including behavioral, electrocortical, and brain imaging paradigms) illustrates that psychopaths have abnormal or weakly lateralized linguistic functions and that their processing of the affective components of language is poor; the deeper affective loading of stimulus material seems to elude them (e.g., Day & Wong, 1996; Hare & Jutai, 1988; Hare & McPherson, 1984; Hare, Williamson, & Harpur, 1988; Intrator et al., 1997; Kiehl et al., 2001; Patrick, 1994; Patrick, Bradley, & Lang, 1993; Patrick, Cuthbert, & Lang, 1994 Williamson, Harpur, & Hare, 1991). Kiehl et al. (2001), for example, found that compared to controls criminal psychopaths showed significantly less affect related activity in the amygdala/hippocampal formation, parahippocampal gyri, ventral striatum and in the anterior and posterior cingulated gyri. Psychopathic criminals also showed evidence of over-activation in the

---

[8] For detailed summaries of this research, see, for instance, Hare (1991, 1996, 1998b), Newman (1998), Newman and Wallace (1993), Wallace, Schmitt, Vitale, and Newman (2000).

bilateral fronto-temporal cortex; with greater activation for affective than for neutral stimuli in the tempora-frontal cortex (Kiehl et al., 2001). These latter data have been interpreted as supporting the notion that psychopathic individuals require more nonlimbic cognitive resources and strategies to process and evaluate affective stimuli that do comparison subjects, presumably due to the absence of appropriate limbic input regarding the affective characteristics (Kiehl et al., 2001). Blair et al. (1997) monitored electrodermal activity (i.e., skin conductance response) of psychopathic and nonpsychopathic subjects during the presentation of threatening and neutral stimuli and reported that psychopathic subjects were hyporesponsive to distress cues (e.g., baby crying) but not to real threat cues (e.g., sight of a snake). Blair et al. (1997) suggested that reduced electrodermal responses to distress cues among psychopathic subjects reflects dysfunction of a violence inhibition mechanism and may account for the psychopath's characteristic lack of empathy. The profound lack of empathy may reflect an inability to generate apt autonomic responses to the pain or distress experienced by another person. Lapierre et al. (1995) found that incarcerated psychopathic individuals were significantly impaired on neuropsychological tasks considered sensitive to orbitofrontal / ventromedial prefrontal dysfunction.[9] They also found that psychopaths did not display performance deficits on measures sensitive to the dorsolateral prefrontal cortex and postero-olandic function.[10]

It is important to note that the neurocognitive impairments that have been found in adult psychopathic individuals are also being found in children with psychopathic tendencies (Blair, 1999; Fisher & Blair, 1998; O'Brien & Frick, 1996). Blair, Colledge, and Mitchell (2001), for example, investigated the performance of boys with psychopathic tendencies and comparison boys, aged 9 to 17 years, on a gambling task (Bechara and colleagues, 1994, 1999) and a learning task (the Intradimensional/Extradimensional (ID/ED) shift task; Dias, Robbins, & Roberts, 1996). The psychopathic boys showed impaired performance on the gambling task but not the ID/ED task, suggesting that psychopathic tendencies reflect amygdala dysfunction.

---

[9] Tasks included a visual go/no go task and the Porteus Maze Test.
[10] Tasks included the Wisconsin Card Sorting Test (WCST) and the Mental Rotation task.

**PREDICTIVE VALIDITY**

*Institutional misbehavior.* It is found that the psychopathy construct has utility in the prediction of disruptive behavior in residential settings in a variety of (mainly North-American) samples of adult male prisoners and forensic psychiatric patients (e.g., Belfrage, Fransson, & Strand , 2000; Buffington-Vollum, Edens, Johnson, & Johnson, 2002; Edens, Buffington-Vollum, Colwell, Johnson, & Johnson, 2002; Gacono, Meloy, Sheppard, Speth, & Roske, 1995; Hare, Clark, Grann, & Thornton, 2000; Hare & McPherson, 1984; Heilbrun et al., 1998; Kosson, Steuerwald, Forth, & Kirkhart, 1997; Kroner & Mills, 2001; Moltó, Poy, & Torrubia, 2000; Pham, Remy, Dailliet, & Lienard, 1998; Reiss, Grubin, & Meux, 1999; Rice, Harris, & Cormier, 1992), female inmates (Salekin, Rogers, & Sewell, 1997), general psychiatric patients (Rasmussen & Levander, 1996), and adolescent offenders (Brandt, Kennedy, Patrick, & Curtin, 1997; Edens, Poythress, & Lilienfeld, 1999; Hicks, Rogers, & Cashel, 2000; Rogers, Johansen, Chang, & Salekin, 1997; Weiler & Widom, 1996). For example, Serin (1991) administered the PCL to 87 male inmates in a medium-security federal prison. The results indicated that the psychopathic inmates (PCL total score ≥ 28) scored higher than the nonpsychopathic inmates on measures of impulsiveness and aggressiveness (Serin, 1991; Serin & Amos, 1991). In addition, he observed that the psychopathic inmates were considerably more abusive, threatening, and violent than the nonpsychopathic inmates. Finally, Serin (1991) noted that the psychopathic prisoners were more likely than the nonpsychopathic inmates to have committed more serious past offenses. Consistent with these findings, Hill, Rogers, and Bickford (1996) found that male adult offenders in a maximum security forensic psychiatric hospital who obtained high scores (i.e., 18 or more) on the PCL:SV were more likely to engage in aggressive and socially disruptive behaviors than individuals with low scores (< 18) on the PCL:SV.[11]

*Recidivism.* Numerous researchers have investigated the ability of the PCL-R to predict recidivism.[12] The results of these research studies generally found that the PCL-R consistently predicted different types (i.e., sexual, violent, general) of recidivism across

---

[11] It is generally recognized that the findings obtained with one version of the PCL are generalizable to the other versions (Hare, 1991).
[12] For extensive (meta-analytic) reviews, see, among others, Hemphill et al. (1998), Salekin, Rogers, and Sewell (1996), Gendreau, Goggin, and Smith (2002) and Walters (2003).

various clinical settings and samples, including male prison inmates or forensic psychiatric patients (e.g., Grann, Långström, Tengström, & Kullgren, 1999; Rice & Harris, 1995a; Serin, 1996; Tengström, Grann, Långström, & Kullgren, 2000), sex offenders (e.g., Barbaree, Seto, Serin, Amos, & Preston, 1994; Furr, 1993; Quinsey, Rice, & Harris, 1995; Rice & Harris, 1997a; Serin, Mailloux, & Malcolm, 2001; Serin, Malcolm, Khanna, & Barbaree, 1994; Wong, 1995), female offenders (Salekin, Rogers, Ustad, & Sewell, 1998), and adolescent (sex) offenders (Forth, Hart, & Hare, 1990; Gretton, McBride, Hare, O'Shaughnessy, & Kumka, 2001; Toupin, Mercier, Déry, Côté, & Hodgins, 1995). The robust association between psychopathy, as measured by the family of Psychopathy Checklists, and future violence is evident even after controlling for traditional risk factors that may confound the relationship (e.g., criminal history and/or demographic characteristics) (Hart, 1998). The results of these studies have led several researchers to address the related question of whether there is a relationship between psychopathy and treatment outcome among institutionalized populations. In the next section we will briefly discuss the small body of empirical research that has addressed this relationship (see also Chapter 6).

*Treatment outcome.* The evaluation of the effectiveness of treatment in reducing (violent) re-offending among (male) adult and adolescent psychopathic individuals has indicated that, in general, those who score high on the PCL-R show a distinctly negative response to treatment (e.g., Harris, Rice, & Quinsey, 1993; Hobson, Shine, & Roberts, 2000; O'Neill, Lidz, & Heilbrun, 2003; Rice, Harris, & Cormier, 1992; Seto & Barbaree, 1999). In one of the earliest studies to address the relationship between (PCL-R) psychopathy and treatment outcome, Ogloff, Wong, and Greenwood (1990) administered the PCL-R to 80 incarcerated male offenders who were participating in a therapeutic community program designed to treat criminal offenders with personality disorders. Ogloff et al. (1990) used the following outcome measures: (1) length of time spent in the therapeutic community program, (2) degree of motivation, and (3) degree of clinical improvement; degree of motivation and degree of clinical improvement were coded from clinical and institutional files. The results indicated that the patients with PCL-R total scores $\geq 27$ were more likely to prematurely terminate participation in the treatment program, showed less motivation and less clinical improvement (Ogloff et al., 1990).

In another study, Rice et al. (1992) found an interaction effect in that *treated* psychopaths recidivated at a *higher* rate (i.e., 77%) than those who did not receive treatment (i.e., 55%) after a 10.5 year follow-up. It should be noted, however, that this treatment program, although considered innovative in the late 1960s and 1970s, was a nontraditional treatment program that "would not meet current ethical standards" (Harris et al, 1991, p. 628). Nevertheless, the findings of Rice et al. (1992) create concern about the involvement of psychopaths in treatment, especially the possibility that participation in certain types of psychological treatment could exacerbate their already high level of violence risk (e.g., see Rice & Harris, 1997b; Yalom, 1995). Further research is needed to determine if the treatment of offenders with (moderate to severe) psychopathy can be made more effective.

## CONCLUSION

Although still a somewhat controversial issue among researchers and clinicians, there seems to be a renewed interest in the concept of psychopathy. It can be concluded from this introductory chapter that operationalization of Cleckley's concept of psychopathy through the development of the PCL-R has served to established its validity. In fact, in the current scientific literature, psychopathy has become virtually synonymous with the PCL-R definition of the construct. As is evident from our review, extensive research with the PCL-R, and its' derivates, over the last 25 years has provided a strong knowledge base regarding the behavioral, interpersonal, and affective characteristics of psychopaths. Specifically, the research suggests that (PCL-R) psychopathy is associated with increased risk of violent and aggressive behavior, disruptive behavior, high rates of (different types of) criminal recidivism, and poor treatment outcome. The PCL-R has become a central tool in risk assessment for future (violent) criminal behavior, not only in its own right (Hemphill et al., 1998; Salekin et al., 1996) but also as an integral feature of a growing body of risk assessment guidelines (e.g., Boer, Hart, Kropp, & Webster, 1997; Borum, 1996; Kropp, Hart, Webster, Eaves, 1994; Webster, Douglas, Eaves, & Hart, 1997; Webster, Eaves, Douglas, & Wintrup, 1995; Webster, Harris, Rice, Cormier, & Quinsey, 1994). Psychopathy is considered a necessary aspect of any thorough examination of future violence risk.

Although the predictive validity of the PCL-R is impressive, caution is warranted in equating dangerousness with psychopathy. Not all violent and dangerous offenders are (PCL-R) psychopaths (Bonta, Harris, Zinger, & Carriere, 1996; Harris, Rice, & Quinsey, 1993; Serin, 1996). Also, claims that the PCL-R should be "the primary instrument ... for appraisals of criminal recidivism and dangerousness" (Hemphill et al., 1998, p. 160) need to be viewed with caution in light of other research. For example, Harris and colleagues (Harris et al., 1993; Rice & Harris, 1997a) identified 11 additional predictors to the PCL-R that, when combined to construct the Violence Risk Appraisal Guide (VRAG; Harris et al., 1993), significantly improved prediction of violent recidivism beyond knowledge of only the PCL-R ($r = .44$ versus $r = .34$). Also, comparisons of the PCL-R with other risk assessment instruments do not always show the PCL-R to be the better predictor. In a recent meta-analysis, Gendreau et al. (2002), for example, found that the Level of Service Inventory-Revised (LSI-R; Andrews & Bonta, 1995) actually performed as well as the PCL-R when the outcome was *violent* recidivism and better than the PCL-R when the outcome was *general* recidivism.

Nevertheless, the research reviewed here indicates that psychopathy is an important factor in understanding and predicting (violent) criminal conduct: "Even those opposed to the very idea of psychopathy cannot ignore its potent explanatory and predictive power — if not as a formal construct, then as a static factor" (Hare, 1998, p. 205).

## MAIN RESEARCH QUESTIONS

Despite the extensive attention that the construct of psychopathy, assessed with the PCL-R, has received from both researchers and clinicians abroad during the past 25 years, surprisingly, no researcher has empirically investigated it's merits in (non)institutionalized populations in the Netherlands. Accordingly, our knowledge is essentially limited to foreign research findings. The necessity of testing the utility of the construct of psychopathy in Dutch forensic psychiatry is therefore evident. Below, the five main research questions addressed in this thesis are outlined:[13]

(1)    What is the reliability and factor structure of the Dutch language version of the Hare Psychopathy Checklist-Revised (PCL-R; Hare, 1991)? (Chapter 3 of this thesis).

Implementation of the PCL-R for clinical use in any new (cultural) context should be accompanied by evaluation of the psychometric status of the instrument in that particular context. The generalizability of the PCL-R's dimensional structure has not yet been established for forensic psychiatric patients in the Netherlands. The study presented in Chapter 3 is designed to examine the (interrater) reliability and factor structure of the Dutch language version of the PCL-R.

(2)    What is the association between psychopathy and DSM-IV Axis I and Axis II disorder? (Chapter 4 of this thesis).

Previous work has generally supported the construct validity of Hare's PCL-R in relation to DSM-III (-R) Axis I and Axis II disorders. Most of this work, however, has involved North American criminal and forensic psychiatric samples. We do not know whether the findings reported are generalizable to Dutch forensic psychiatric patients. Also, to the best of our knowledge, no study has been published that systematically examined the association between PCL-R psychopathy and Axis I and Axis II disorders of the last edition of the Diagnostic and Statistical Manual of Mental Disorders (DSM-IV; American Psychiatric Association, 1994). Chapter 4 describes a study that was designed to examine the association between PCL-R psychopathy and (1) assessment of DSM-IV Axis I disorders and (2) DSM-III-R/DSM-IV Axis II disorders.

(3)    What is the predictive power of psychopathy in relation to inpatient disruptive behavior? (Chapter 5 of this thesis).

---

[13] In order to avoid redundancy, it was decided not to provide an extensive description of the specific research questions or hypotheses. or more detailed background information on the hypotheses, see the introductory paragraph of the separate studies presented in Chapters 3 through 7.

Studies have demonstrated numerous risk factors to be associated with inpatient violence in (forensic) psychiatric patients, including individual (e.g., age, number of total prior convictions, psychotic disorder, drug/alcohol abuse) and situational (e.g., overcrowding, staff inexperience, tolerance of violence) factors. While research that addresses the association between psychopathy and inpatient disruptive behavior is rapidly expanding, only a handful of studies have examined this relationship in forensic psychiatric patients. In Chapter 5, a prospective study examining the strength of the association between PCL-R psychopathy and various forms of disruptive behavior in a residential forensic psychiatric setting is presented.

(4)     What is the relationship between psychopathy and change in dynamic risk factors during forensic psychiatric treatment? (Chapter 6 of this thesis).

Effective treatment to reduce recidivism requires the targeting of appropriate dynamic risk factors (e.g., Andrews, Bonta, & Hoge, 1990; Andrews & Bonta, 2003). Risk factors can be *static* or *dynamic*. Static risk factors are those that are unlikely to change, such as sex and prior offenses and are not suitable as treatment targets. Dynamic risk factors, on the other hand, are characteristics which are amenable to change, and when changed, are expected to result in a corresponding decrease (or increase) in recidivism risk. The main objective of the study presented in Chapter 6 is to investigate the relationship between PCL-R psychopathy as a trait and change in relevant dynamic risk factors during forensic psychiatric treatment.

(5)     Do rapists identified as psychopathic recidivate more frequently and sooner than nonpsychopathic rapists following the termination of treatment (Chapter 7 of this thesis).

The identification of risk factors that are associated with recidivism in sex offenders plays an important role in determining effective risk management strategies. The main objective of the retrospective study presented in Chapter 7 is to investigate the role of PCL-R psychopathy as a risk factor for re-offending in a sample of sex offenders, convicted for rape or sexual assault, who had returned to society after (intensive) forensic psychiatric treatment. The second goal of the study is to examine the degree to which a combination of PCL-R psychopathy and sexual deviance can predict sexual recidivism.

## SETTING

The setting of the research reported in this thesis is the Dr. Henri van der Hoeven Kliniek, located in Utrecht, and one of the 13 forensic psychiatric institutions in the Netherlands. To give the reader an impression of the treatment process and its different stages, the procedures in the Dr. Henri van der Hoeven Kliniek will be described in some detail here — with special reference to psychological assessment procedures used to periodically evaluate treatment progress.

### TREATMENT MODEL

The Dr. Henri van der Hoeven Kliniek is a 135-bed forensic psychiatric hospital for the treatment of mentally disordered offenders who have been sentenced by criminal court to involuntary commitment because of (severely) diminished responsibility for the offense(s) they committed. In terms of legal status, most patients are sentenced to a 'maatregel van terbeschikkingstelling' (TBS-order), a judicial measure which can be translated as 'disposal to be treated on behalf of the state' (for a discussion of the TBS-order, see Chapter 2). The purpose of the TBS-order is to protect society from offenders with unacceptably high risks of recidivism, directly through involuntary admission to a secure forensic psychiatric hospital, and indirectly through the treatment provided there.

The hospital as a whole is organized as a therapeutic community. A central concept in the treatment model is the stimulation of the patient's awareness that he is responsible for his own life, including his offenses and his progress in treatment. This premise is basic to the way the hospital is organized and to all treatment activities. Patients reside in living groups of circa 10 patients, where they can develop and practice alternative styles and skills. An adequately functioning social network in the outside world is considered important to support the patient during treatment and after termination during his reintegration into society. Treatment progress is evaluated every three months by the treatment team, which includes the supervising psychologist, group leaders, the psychotherapist and the social worker of the patient.

The general treatment model of the Dr. Henri van der Hoeven Kliniek is eclectic with an emphasis on diminishing violence risk through interventions aimed at increasing the patient's insight and control over his behavior. To this end, a treatment program is constructed, composed of individual and/or group psychotherapy, job training, education, creative arts and sports. Patients participate in various group therapy programs, such as social skills training, aggression and impulsivity management. There are special programs for substance abusers and sex offenders. Almost all patients receive individual psychotherapy, which is cognitive-behavioral, with an integration of several approaches, such as Young's (1994) cognitive therapy for personality disorders, Linehan's (1993) dialectical behavior therapy and the offense script and relapse prevention method (Laws, 1989; see also van Beek, 1999).

## OBSERVATION AND ASSESSMENT

The first two months of the patients' stay at the hospital are used for observation, assessment and preparation for treatment. From the first day on, the patient has a program of daily activities, including work, education, creative arts and sports. Work supervisors and teachers observe patients during their activities and report their observations. The patient also spends time at his living group (see below), where group leaders make observations during structured and unstructured activities.

During this period, psychologists see the patient for personality assessment. The objective of personality assessment is to obtain insight into the factors that are related to the patient's violence risk. To this end, a standard test battery, including semi-structured interviews (for DSM-IV Axis II disorders and the Psychopathy Checklist-Revised interview), self-report personality inventories [e.g., the Minnesota Multiphasic Personality Inventory-2 (MMPI-2; Butcher, Dahlstrom, Graham, Tellegen, & Kaemmer, 1989; Butcher, Graham, Ben-Porath, Tellegen, & Kaemmer, 2001) and anger, impulsivity and interpersonal behavior scales] and indirect tests (e.g., the Rorschach Inkblot Method; Exner, 1993) is administered (T1) (see also Hildebrand & de Ruiter, 1999). *Multimethod* assessment is recommended, because distinct assessment methods provide unique sources of data (Meyer et al., 2000) and results from separate instruments can be used to crossvalidate each other (see also Chapter 6). Furthermore, the use of psychometric instruments is to assess the extent to which a patients has changed during the treatment, or to examine the effectiveness of recommendations and interventions. Initial pretreatment assessments in conjunction with need assessments should identify which criminogenic factors (see Chapter 6) needed to be addressed in treatment. Also, structured clinical guidelines for the assessment of violence risk (HCR-20; Webster et al., 1997) and sexual violence risk (SVR-20; Boer et al., 1997) are administered. By using standardized risk assessment instruments, the appraisal of offense risk gains in standardization, transparency, and empirical support (Webster et al., 1997). Table 5 presents the assessment instruments used in the Dr. Henri van der Hoeven Kliniek.

**TABLE 5**
*Forensic Psychological Test Battery used in the Dr. Henri van der Hoeven Kliniek*

| Domain | Instruments |
|---|---|
| Risk of future violence | HCR-20; SVR-20 |
| Impulsivity | BIS-11; MMPI-2; PCL-R; RIM CS |
| Interpersonal behavior | ICL-R; MMPI-2; RIM CS |
| Personality structure / - disorders | MMPI-2; RIM CS; SIDP-IV |
| Psychopathy | PCL-R |
| Substance use problems | PCL-R; MMPI-2 |
| Anger / anger control | MMPI-2; NAS; PCL-R; RIM CS |

*Note.* BIS-11 = *Barratt Impulsiveness Scale* (Barratt, 1994); HCR-20 = *Historical, Clinical, Risk Management-20* (Webster et al., 1997); ICL-R = *Interpersonal Checklist-Revised* (LaForge & Suczek, 1955); MMPI-2 = *Minnesota Multiphasic Personality Inventory* (Butcher et al., 1989); NAS = *Novaco Anger Scale* (Novaco, 1994); PCL-R = *Psychopathy Checklist-Revised* (Hare, 1991); RIM CS = Rorschach Inkblot Method, applied according to Exner's *Comprehensive System* (Exner, 1993); SIDP-IV = *Structured Interview for DSM-IV Personality Disorders* (Pfohl, Blum, & Zimmerman, 1994); SVR-20 = Sexual Violence Risk-20 (Boer et al., 1997).

During the first weeks, the patient also meets with one of the psychotherapists and with the social worker who is assigned to his living group. These sessions are scheduled to determine what role psychotherapy and the patient's social network could have in his treatment. The observation and assessment period ends with the so-called "treatment indication meeting", a staff meeting where all hospital staff and the patient convene to discuss the core problems of the patient and his treatment plan.

## THE LIVING GROUP

Most patients reside in a living group, where they live with fellow-patients in a kind of 'house'. Every living group consists of 8 to 10 patients, supervised by group leaders. Daily life in the group provides patients with experiences that have to do with sharing responsibilities, social skills and spending leisure time. Each patient has his own room. The treatment team consists of a supervising psychologist, a social worker and the group leaders and is responsible for planning, progress and evaluation of the patient's treatment. The group leaders have a diversity of tasks: they are present at meals and at group discussions; they supervise the structure of daily life; they write treatment plans and daily logs of their experiences with patients.

The hospital has a special ward for individual treatment, where patients who are unsuitable for placement in a regular living group are admitted. In general, the goal is to replace patients in a regular living group after a period of intensive individual treatment, but this objective is not always met. Since the beginning of the 1990's, there is a special living group for patients with psychotic disorders. This group is more structured and less demanding; medication adherence and psycho-education are the most important aspects of the treatment here.

## TREATMENT EVALUATION

Treatment progress is evaluated every three months, both orally and in writing. The patient's progress is discussed with fellow patients during a meeting with the living group and during a meeting with the persons (teachers, therapists, work supervisors, etc.) involved in the patient's treatment. All patients in our hospital are re-tested 18-24 months after admission (T2) with *a number* of the personality tests that were administered upon admission to the hospital, and again 42 months after admission (T3). In this way, objective instruments provide information on the patient's progress. The 'what works' literature (e.g., Andrews, 1995) highlights the importance of having evaluation procedures built into programs to check they are meeting the stated objectives as part of a continuous review process. In addition, behavior change (the ultimate goal) is not expected to occur in a vacuum: concomitant changes in personality, beliefs, and attitudes are expected.

Important phases in the treatment process are discussed at evaluations. Subsequently, the patient may be invited to submit a proposal for extension of leave, which needs to include the reasons why he thinks he has changed so that extended leave is warranted. Such a proposal is discussed in the patient's living group, in the treatment team and in the so-called 'Hospital council', which consists of staff members and patient representatives from all living groups. The Hospital council meets every day and serves to maintain a safe and viable therapeutic milieu through cooperation between staff members and patients. After the patient's proposal has been discussed in all these organs, the final decision about extension of leave is made in the general hospital staff meeting.

**RESOCIALIZATION/AFTERCARE**

The hospital aims to limit the duration of the inpatient treatment phase for each patient, of course without losing sight of society's safety. When feasible, a patient is placed in a so-called 'transmural setting'. 'Transmuralization' is an intensive resocialization program whereby patients are supported by a special ambulatory team of group leaders, who supervise them during this resocialization phase. They monitor and assist patients in their own living environment. Patients can be re-admitted to the hospital in case there are signs of becoming a risk to society. There are several types of transmural settings:

(1)    Supervised living in apartments owned by the hospital or in rental apartments. Characteristic of this type of forensic supervised living is regular contact between the patient and staff members of the hospital, but there is no 24-hour supervision. The patient's daily life mainly takes place outside the walls of the hospital, although in some cases he may visit the hospital almost daily, for example to see his psychotherapist or to go to work training;

(2)    Collaboration with a sheltered housing organization in the city of Utrecht.
        Since 1991, the hospital has the possibility to place patients with limited social and cognitive capacities (who realize sufficiently that they will need supervision for an extended period of time) in sheltered housing. Most of these patients follow a treatment program inside the hospital during the day. After a certain period, their

activities inside the hospital are often replaced by activities in society, such as volunteer work or a paid job in a welfare facility;

(3)     Clinical admission to a forensic ward of a general psychiatric hospital. For patients who have insufficient capacities to support themselves in a sheltered living arrangement, the Dr. Henri van der Hoeven Kliniek has a number of beds in a general psychiatric hospital. These patients may suffer from psychoses which cannot be managed adequately with medication or they may be unable to adhere to their medication regimen without intensive external supervision. They need long term, clinical treatment to prevent psychotic decompensation.

CHAPTER 2

TREATMENT

UNDER THE DUTCH TBS-ORDER[1]

[1] Parts of this chapter are based on:
Ruiter, C. de, & Hildebrand, M. (2003). The dual nature of forensic psychiatric practice: Risk assessment and management under the Dutch TBS-order. In P.J. van Koppen & S.D. Penrod (Eds.), *Adversarial versus inquisitorial justice: Psychological perspectives on criminal justice systems* (pp. 91-106). New York: Kluwer/Plenum.

## SUMMARY

In this chapter, we briefly describe a special provision in the Dutch criminal code that allows for a period of mandatory treatment following a prison sentence for mentally disordered offenders: *Terbeschikkingstelling* (TBS-order). The purpose of TBS is to protect society from unacceptably high risks of recidivism, directly through involuntary admission to a forensic psychiatric hospital, and indirectly through the treatment provided there. Theoretically, treatment under the TBS-order is of indefinite duration if the offender continues to pose a risk to society. Every one or two years the court re-evaluates the patient in order to determine whether the risk of (violent) recidivism is still too high and treatment needs to be continued. The legal criteria of the TBS-order are described, the important issue of violent risk assessment/management is touched upon, and treatment effectiveness research is reported. Finally, some strengths and weaknesses of forensic psychiatric practice under the TBS-order in the Netherlands are discussed.

# INTRODUCTION

Mentally disordered or personality disordered offenders are often envisioned as individuals who violently, unexpectedly, and without reason attack innocent victims. Moreover, the system supposedly treating them is seen as neither reducing the likelihood of future danger nor as protecting society from it. For others, however, mentally/personality disordered offenders trigger sympathy as victims of impulses over which they have little control and as caught in a system they do not understand, which fails to respond to their unique needs. When a (released) forensic psychiatric patient commits a violent crime, the public becomes strongly polarized against the forensic mental health system. To facilitate understanding the movement of this category of offenders through the (Dutch) criminal justice system to the forensic hospital system, the Dutch situation for making decisions regarding mentally disordered or personality disordered offenders is described in a nutshell.[2]

# LEGAL REGULATION

According to the Dutch Code of Criminal Procedure (CCP; *Wetboek van Strafvordering*, Sv., Article 352, Section 2) and the Dutch Code of Criminal Law (CCL; *Wetboek van Strafrecht*, Sr., Article 39), as a general rule, in cases where the criminal act is proven but the offender cannot be held responsible, because of a mental disorder or defect, the offender will not be sentenced but discharged.[3] The question whether the defendant has committed the offense precedes and is distinguished from the question whether he[4] is punishable, which depends (among other things) on whether the defendant is to be held responsible for the crime he committed (see Article 350 Sv.)

Dutch criminal law recognizes two measures that can be applied to mentally disturbed offenders. First, the law offers the possibility for a defendant who is found not responsible for the crime, to be admitted to a psychiatric hospital, but only if he is a danger to himself or to others or to the general safety of persons or property (Art. 37, section 1

---

[2] For more detailed descriptions on the assessment and treatment of mentally disordered offenders in the Netherlands, see Malsch and Hielkema (1999), van Marle (2002), de Ruiter and Hildebrand (2003).

[3] In Dutch terminology: *ontslagen van alle rechtsvervolging*.

[4] The male pronoun is used in this and the following chapters for referring to either gender.

CCL). Second, Article 37a of the Dutch CCL states that a defendant who, at the time of the alleged crime, suffered from a mental defect or disorder may receive what is called a 'disposal to be involuntarily admitted to a forensic psychiatric hospital on behalf of the state' (*maatregel van terbeschikkingstelling, TBS*-order). The Dutch Ministry of Justice states that the legitimacy of the TBS order lies in the right for society to protect itself against unacceptable risks of (severe) criminal behavior. The nature of the order is not intended as retribution or to cause suffering but to provide custodial care aimed at motivating the offender to undergo treatment.

The law requires that *at least* two experts from different disciplines report on the defendant before the trial court can decide to impose a TBS-order. One of the experts must be a psychiatrist (Art. 37a, Section 3 and Art. 37, Section 2 Sr.). A TBS-order can be imposed by the court if the following three conditions apply (Art. 37a Sr.):

(1)     The defendant must suffer from a mental disorder, which means that his responsibility for the alleged crime is (severely) diminished or absent.
        The basic assumption is that each defendant is fully responsible for all of his acts. In case of a disorder, the court will decide on the basis of reports by behavioral experts *to what extent* this disorder has influenced the behavior of the defendant at the moment of the alleged crime;

(2)     The crime carries a prison sentence of at least four years, or the offense belongs to a category of offenses specifically mentioned in the law, although carrying a lesser sentence;

(3)     There is a risk for the safety of persons or for the general safety of persons or goods.[5]

Article 37a of the (old) Dutch Code of Criminal Law created the possibility of diminished responsibility. On the basis of this, more refined 'levels' of criminal responsibility were introduced in the Dutch jurisprudence, and eventually a five-point

---

[5] Thus, diminished responsibility does not always result in the recommendation and the imposition of involuntarily admission to a forensic hospital under the TBS-order. Only in cases where, in addition to a mental disorder being established, it is judged that the person is *at risk to commit another serious (sexually) violent crime in the future*, an involuntary admission to a forensic psychiatric hospital will be imposed.

sliding scale emerged, indicating the degree of criminal responsibility: full, slightly diminished, diminished, severely diminished, and total absence of responsibility. In case of diminished responsibility, the judge may sentence a prison term for that part of his psychological functioning for which the defendant had freedom of choice (i.e., the choice not to commit the offense). Consequently, offenders considered to have diminished responsibility for the crimes they committed can (and most of the time will) also be sentenced to imprisonment. The decision by the court to direct both a sentence and involuntary admission is based on the consideration that a combination of the two is a more effective instrument in achieving protection than involuntary admission to a forensic hospital on its own. If a person is sentenced to a long penal sanction in conjunction with involuntary admission to a forensic hospital, the prison sentence is executed first; after the offender has served his sentence he will be transferred to a forensic hospital.

The combination of imprisonment and involuntary admission to a forensic psychiatric hospital poses significant ethical questions. The TBS is ordered to allow treatment of the psychiatric disorder of the offender and therefore there is an ethical obligation to admit the patient to a hospital as soon as possible. From a medical point of view, one can argue that it is ethically unjust to postpone the treatment the patient needs, i.e., by executing the prison sentence first. On the other hand, it seems also ethically unjust to treat the patient first, and execute the prison sentence after he is successfully treated and no longer considered a danger to society.

Theoretically, a TBS-order is of indefinite duration (Art. 38e, Section 2 Sr.). Initially imposed for two years (Art. 38d, Section 1 Sr.), it may be extended for one or two year periods of time as the court re-evaluates the patient to determine whether the risk for the safety of (other) people or for the general safety of persons or goods is still too high (Art. 38d, Section 2 Sr.). Most of the time, TBS involves involuntary admission to a specialized maximum security forensic psychiatric hospital (Art. 37d, Section 1 Sr.) aimed at motivating the patient to participate in the treatment programs offered by the hospital. The implication for clinical practice is that it is legally permitted to place a patient in a living group with fellow patients and to structure his daily life in such a way that it is almost impossible for him to avoid contact with members of the hospital staff (e.g., sociotherapists). Neither on ethical nor on legal grounds can there be an escape from the obligation to participate in a therapeutic milieu in order to facilitate social contacts aimed at motivating the patient for treatment. However, patients are free to refuse, for example, pharmacotherapy and to avoid participating in specific therapeutic activities such as psychotherapy.[6] As a rule, compulsory treatment is only possible if patients are a threat to themselves or other people. Although there are differences in the treatment models the Dutch forensic psychiatric hospitals adhere to, the treatment provided within the legal framework of the TBS generally strives to effect structural behavioral change that leads to a reduction in violence risk.

Every forensic psychiatric hospital has a legal obligation to provide (1) security to society; (2) treatment for the offender-patient, and (3) to protect the civil rights of the latter. These components need to be balanced in the forensic psychiatric setting, and each hospital makes its own choices in this regard, in conjunction with its therapeutic framework and security level. Although the treatment models of the forensic psychiatric institutions in the Netherlands vary, they all involve a composite of education, work training, individual and group psychotherapy, creative arts and sports activities.

A relatively new development is *transmuralization*: An intensive resocialization program whereby patients are supported by a special ambulatory team of group leaders, who supervise them during this resocialization phase (see also Chapter 1). They monitor and assist patients in their own living environment. Patients can be re-admitted to the hospital in case there are signs of becoming a risk to society.

## VIOLENCE RISK ASSESSMENT AND MANAGEMENT

Risk assessment/management is an ongoing task of the staff of forensic psychiatric hospitals where TBS patients stay. All proposals for extensions of leave have to be announced to the Ministry of Justice, who carries the ultimate responsibility for the execution of the TBS order. The Ministry has the right to raise objections to the leave proposals submitted by the hospitals, and withholds permission in some cases. Leave decisions that have to be approved include: the first time the TBS patient is allowed outside the physical security of the institution, still under staff supervision; travel without staff supervision; leave on probation.

---

[6] Because of the fact that the TBS-order can be extended as long as the TBS-patient poses a risk, refusal of treatment generally implies a prolonged stay in the hospital.

Every one or two years, the court (Art. 38d, Section 1 Sr.) reviews the patient's case, and decides whether the TBS needs to be extended or can be terminated. The hospital has to submit a report to the court providing information on the mental disorder of the patient, treatment progress, assessment of recidivism risk, and advice on the extension or termination of the TBS. The court does not always follow the hospital's advice. In a long-term (> 5 years) follow-up of 40 patients who had been treated at the Dr. Henri van der Hoeven Kliniek, recidivism rates of patients who had been released by the judge, against the hospital's advice, were notably higher than recidivism rates of patients released on the hospital's advice (25% vs. 55% for serious recidivism that resulted in unconditional imprisonment and/or TBS; Niemantsverdriet, 1993). Similar findings are reported by Van Emmerik (1989) and Leuw (1999).

After a patient has been detained under the TBS order for six years, the law (Art. 509, Section 4 Sv.) requires two independent behavioral experts, a psychologist and a psychiatrist, to submit an independent forensic report to inform the court about the mental disorder and the risk of recidivism of the patient. The court then decides about extension or termination of the TBS order on the basis of the report provided by the hospital where the patient is being treated and those of the two independent experts. This so-called 6-years procedure is to safeguard the patient from the well-known biases that treatment staff are liable to when they have to assess future violence risk in their own patients (Dernevik, 1999).

## TREATMENT EFFECTIVENESS RESEARCH

Although the TBS order was introduced in the criminal justice system in 1928, research into the effectiveness of the treatments offered in the Dutch forensic psychiatric hospitals is rather scarce. Unfortunately, there are no adequate outcome studies of the TBS system, so it is difficult to know whether it works or not (McInerny, 2000). A number of follow-up studies of different patient cohorts from 1974 through 1993, have documented serious violent recidivism rates between 15 and 20% over follow-up periods of three to eight years for patients for whom the TBS order was terminated (van Emmerik, 1985, 1989; Leuw, 1995, 1999). Unfortunately, there is currently no research evidence showing that (reduced) recidivism is related to treatment process and/or outcome. A 2-year cross-sectional follow-up study of 59 personality disordered patients, during their inpatient treatment in the Dr. Henri van der Hoeven Kliniek, demonstrated that 25% of these patients changed reliably and to a clinically significant degree on a number of self-report measures of personality and psychopathology (Greeven, 1997). The overall personality structure of the patients, however, remained essentially the same, and it remains to be seen how these patients will fare after they have been released into society.

## STRENGTHS AND WEAKNESSES

The Dutch criminal justice system provides a number of legal procedures that offer possibilities for a unique way of risk assessment, management and treatment for mentally disordered offenders. The TBS order, with its focus on therapeutic milieu treatment and opportunities for education and work training, offers mentally disordered offenders an opportunity towards resocialization and rehabilitation, which is in sharp contrast to the way North American criminal justice systems deal with this group of offenders.

Still, there are a number of shortcomings in current forensic psychiatric practice in the Netherlands that need improvement in the coming years. First, the treatments provided under the TBS order are not evidence-based (see de Ruiter, 2003), and treatment methods have failed to keep pace with those of general psychiatry (van Marle, 2002). In the words of McInerny (2000), "treatment (...) appeared to be on an *ad hoc* basis, with little adherence to the principles of evidence-based medicine. Consequently, TBS patients are not, in my view, receiving adequate assessment and treatment" (p. 226).

There have not been any studies that examine the relation between treatment outcome and recidivism, which is a prerequisite for determining the effectiveness of the TBS measure. Moreover, there is no information on the differential effectiveness of the treatments provided, i.e., whether treatment is successful with some types of patients but not with others. Also, there is insufficient knowledge about the decision making process for termination of the TBS-order with acceptable risk for society. To date, the most widely used method in forensic practice, at least in the Netherlands, is the unstructured clinical judgment approach that is exclusively based on the professional expertise of the clinicians. Research, however, has revealed several limitations of the unstructured clinical judgment approach, such as poor reliability and validity (Monahan, 1981).[7] For this reason, several scholars have recommended to employ structured risk assessment procedures in order to optimize accuracy and validity (e.g., Borum, 1996; Webster, Douglas, Eaves, & Hart, 1997). However, risk assessments conducted in the Dutch forensic psychiatric hospitals are generally based on (behavioral) observations by treatment staff in different roles and from different professions (nurses, teachers, work supervisors, psychotherapists, etc.). The psychologist or psychiatrist who carries the ultimate treatment responsibility for an individual patient integrates these observations and provides the court with a description and evaluation of the patients' treatment and states the opinion of the hospital staff about the risk of recidivism. *Standardized* risk assessments, based on psychological testing procedures (e.g., the PCL-R; Hare, 1991) and structured clinical guidelines for risk assessment (e.g., the HCR-20; Webster et al., 1997), conducted by *independent* assessors, are, unfortunately, not yet general practice in Dutch forensic psychiatric hospitals.

Second, growing criticism by politicians, the media and the lay public on the expensive 'TBS system' serves to foster long overdue reconsideration of current practices. Few forensic behavioral experts make use of structured risk assessment instruments, which have been proven to be more reliable and valid than unstructured clinical judgment (Grove & Meehl, 1996; Webster et al., 1997).

To conclude, empirically grounded research is needed to improve assessment and prediction of the risk of recidivism and to provide an evidence-base for treatment programs so hopefully in the future recidivism rates will be brought further down. The studies presented in this thesis are an attempt to contribute to this empirical research base.

---

[7] For a discussion of these limitations, see Quinsey, Harris, Rice, and Cormier (1998). For a detailed discussion about the clinical-actuarial approach controversy, the reader is referred to Douglas, Cox, and Webster (1999) and Litwack (2001).

Chapter 3


# RELIABILITY AND FACTOR STRUCTURE

# OF THE DUTCH LANGUAGE VERSION OF THE

# HARE PSYCHOPATHY CHECKLIST-REVISED[1]

[1] A slightly different version of this chapter was published as:
Hildebrand, M., Ruiter, C., de, Vogel, V., de, & Wolf, P., van der (2002). Reliability and factor structure of the Dutch language version of Hare's Psychopathy Checklist-Revised. *International Journal of Forensic Mental Health*, *1*, 139-154.
We appreciate the input of Gerard H. Maassen, Stephen D. Hart, and an anonymous reviewer, who commented on previous versions of this chapter.

## SUMMARY

The interrater and internal reliability and factor structure of the Dutch language version of the Psychopathy Checklist-Revised (PCL-R; Hare, 1991) was examined in a mixed sample of 107 forensic psychiatric patients. In addition, the potential role of two different information sources, real-life interview versus videotaped interview, when scoring the PCL-R, was evaluated. Interrater reliabilities of individual items and the PCL-R total score were good to excellent. Good agreement on the categorical diagnosis of psychopathy was also obtained (weighted Cohen's $\kappa$ = .63 for simultaneous comparison of three raters). The internal consistency of the PCL-R was found to be high, as indicated by a Cronbach's alpha of 0.87, with an alpha of 0.83 for both Factor 1 and Factor 2. Comparisons between real-life and videotaped interview demonstrated that the information source did not influence the raters' coding. Confirmatory factor analysis (CFA) indicated that the two-factor structure obtained by Hare (1991) in the standardization samples did not fit the current data well. CFA also failed to confirm the three-factor model identified by Cooke and Michie (2001). Exploratory principal components analysis extracted two main factors, which accounted for 44% of the variance. It is concluded that the Dutch language version of the PCL-R can be reliably rated by trained professionals, its factor structure resembles the traditional two-factor model to some extent, and future research should include larger samples of different populations such as prisoners and general psychiatric patients.

## INTRODUCTION

Psychopathy is a controversial psychiatric concept (e.g., Lewis, 1974). Definitions of the term psychopathy have historically been both diverse and difficult to operationalize (e.g., Craft, 1965; Dolan & Coid, 1993; Hare, 1970; McCord & McCord, 1964), and research on psychopathy has been characterized by the absence of a clear and generally agreed upon conceptualization of the disorder (O'Kane, Fawcett, & Blackburn, 1996). Despite the fact that the concept of psychopathy has been obscured by a multitude of definitions, the clinical description of psychopathy provided by Cleckley (1941/1982) has received widespread acceptance among contemporary researchers and clinicians. Cleckley provided the first systematic clinical account of psychopathy, defining psychopathy as a constellation of 16 personality traits, reflecting both the affective and interpersonal characteristics that have traditionally been considered central to psychopathy, including egocentricity, failure to form close emotional bonds, callousness, and lack of guilt.

Much of the recent interest in the construct of psychopathy is attributable to the development of the Hare Psychopathy Checklist-Revised (PCL-R; Hare, 1991) and its ability to predict future (violent) criminal behavior (e.g., Hart, 1998; Hemphill, Hare, & Wong, 1998; Salekin, Rogers, & Sewell, 1996). Hare (1980), by adapting components of Cleckley's conceptualization of psychopathy, and adding items related to antisocial behavior, developed and validated the Psychopathy Checklist (PCL), followed by a revised version, the PCL-R (Hare, 1991). The PCL-R is a 20-item clinical construct scale completed on the basis of a semi-structured interview and file information. Items are scored on a three point scale (0 = *item does not apply*, 1 = *item applies to a certain extent*, 2 = *item definitely applies*). The total score can range from 0 to 40, reflecting the degree to which an individual resembles the prototypical psychopath.

The Hare PCL-R was initially developed and validated with data from North American samples of male adult offenders and forensic psychiatric patients. A growing body of research has demonstrated the reliability and validity of the PCL-R for prison and forensic psychiatric samples in other countries (e.g., Grann, Långström, Tengström, & Stålenheim, 1998; Moltó, Poy, & Torrubia, 2000; Tengström, Grann, Långström, & Kullgren, 2000). In addition, reliability and validity studies with adolescent offenders

(Brandt, Kennedy, Patrick, & Curtin, 1997; Forth & Burke, 1998; Forth & Mailloux, 2000), substance abusers (e.g., Alterman, Caccioloa, & Rutherford, 1993; Rutherford, Cacciola, Alterman, & McKay, 1996), female offenders (Salekin, Rogers, & Sewell, 1997), and even male and female non-criminals (Forth, Brown, Hart & Hare, 1996) have been conducted.

At least initially, factor analytic studies of the PCL (Haapasalo & Pulkkinnen, 1992; Harpur, Hare, & Hakstian, 1989; Harpur, Hakstian, & Hare, 1988; Templeman & Wong, 1984) and the PCL-R (e.g., Cooke, 1995; Hare, 1991; Hare et al., 1990; Hobson & Shine, 1998; Windle & Dumenci, 1999) showed that PCL(-R) psychopathy is a higher order clinical construct composed of two distinct and moderately correlated factors. PCL-R Factor 1 consists of a cluster of eight items reflecting the affective and interpersonal features (core personality traits) of psychopathy, and has been labeled "Selfish, callous and remorseless use of others" (Hare, 1991; Hare, Harpur et al., 1990). Factor 2 consists of nine items reflecting the social deviance features of psychopathy and has been labeled "Chronically unstable and antisocial lifestyle." The remaining three items of the PCL-R (promiscuous sexual behavior, many short-term marital relationships and criminal versatility) did not load on either factor (Hare, 1991; Hare, Harpur et al., 1990). Difficulty replicating the initial two-factor solution, however, has occurred in a number of selected samples, including female offenders (Salekin, Rogers, & Sewell, 1997), African-American offenders (Kosson, Smith, & Newman, 1990), a mixed sample of community- and prison-based methadone patients (Darke, Kay, Finley-Jones, & Hall, 1998), and a large sample of substance-dependent male and female patients (McDermott et al., 2000). Furthermore, various researchers have proposed alternative conceptualizations of dimensions that might underlie the PCL and PCL-R (Darke et al., 1998; Haapasalo & Pulkkinnen, 1992; Raine, 1985). Recently, Cooke and Michie (2001) reexamined the adequacy of the two-factor model of psychopathy. They arrived at the conclusion that "although the two-factor model has served as a useful heuristic device to guide research on psychopathy, it does not provide an adequate structural model for psychopathy" (p. 173). Using confirmatory factor analysis, Cooke and Michie (2001) identified a three-factor hierarchical model, based on 13 of the 20 PCL-R items, in which a coherent superordinate factor (i.e., psychopathy), was underpinned by an interpersonal (*Deceitful interpersonal style*), affective (*Deficient affective experience*), and behavioral (*Impulsive and irresponsible behavioral style*) factor. Contrary to the two-factor model, the three-factor model places little emphasis on criminality.

## THE PRESENT STUDY

Implementation of the PCL-R for clinical use in any new (cultural) context should be accompanied by a thorough evaluation of the psychometric status of the instrument in that particular context. According to the cross-cultural literature, this should include examining of structural invariance (via confirmatory factor analysis) and metric invariance (via item respons theory or differential item functioning; e.g., Cooke, Kosson, & Michie, 2001; van de Vijver & Leung, 1997). Different offender populations require separate norms and validity data, because findings from one sample may not be applicable to another. In the case of adoption of an instrument (i.e., the PCL-R) from one cultural group to another, one is interested in adopting the nomological network of the underlying construct tapped by the instrument, as established in the original culture. Relevant to the issue of cross-cultural adaptation, this nomological network can be understood as based on two sets of relationship: (1) the internal network of empirical relationships within the factor structure of the assessment instrument, and (2) the relationship of the instrument to external correlates associated with the construct of interest (Ben-Porath, 1990). To establish the cross-cultural validity of the PCL-R, both internal and external sets of relationships must be demonstrated to be invariant across cultural (or ethnic) groups. Approaches based on classical test theory have limited value in this regard (e.g., van de Vijver & Leung, 1997). Cross validation of the factor structure across groups using confirmatory factor analytic techniques and item response theory (IRT) modeling (Cooke & Michie, 1997; Cooke, Michie, Hart, & Hare, 1999), for example, have become widely used in psychological assessment research as a way to study the underlying structure of the data.

The generalizability of the PCL-R's dimensional structure has not yet been established for forensic psychiatric patients in the Netherlands. The present study was designed to examine the reliability and factor structure of the Dutch language version of the PCL-R in a sample of forensic psychiatric patients involuntarily admitted to the Dr. Henri van der Hoeven Kliniek, a forensic psychiatric hospital in the Netherlands. First, we examine the interrater reliability of PCL-R item and total scores as well as the internal reliability (item homogeneity and internal consistency) of the PCL-R. In addition, we examine the role of two different information sources in rating the PCL-R. Hare (personal communication, October 1997) suggested that different information sources (i.e., real-life interview versus videotaped interview) might play a role in the scoring of the PCL-R. Face-to-face interactions in a real-life interview might result in different general impressions, and thus different scores, than impressions based on videotaped interviews. Particularly scores on PCL-R items pertaining to essentially "soft" or "impressionistic" data (Cooke, 1995, p. 111), such as Item 1 (*Glibness/superficial charm*), Item 5 (*Conning/manipulative*) or Item 7 (*Shallow affect*) may be more susceptible to a possible source effect, because they require a considerable degree of subjective judgment. Finally, we examine the factor structure of the Dutch language version of the PCL-R.

## METHOD

### SETTING

The study was conducted at the Dr. Henri van der Hoeven Kliniek, a ± 135-bed forensic psychiatric hospital for the residential treatment of mentally disordered offenders who are sentenced by criminal court to involuntary commitment because of (severely) diminished responsibility for the offense(s) they committed. In terms of legal status, most patients admitted to our hospital are sentenced by criminal court to a '*maatregel van terbeschikkingstelling*' (TBS-order), a judicial measure which can be translated as 'disposal to be treated on behalf of the state'. The purpose of the TBS-order is to protect society from unacceptably high risks of recidivism, directly through involuntary admission to a forensic psychiatric hospital, and indirectly through the treatment provided there. Every one or two years the court re-evaluates the patient in order to determine whether the risk of (violent) recidivism is still too high and treatment needs to be continued. Theoretically, treatment under the TBS-order is of indefinite duration if the offender continues to pose a risk to society. (For discussions of TBS, see van Marle, 2002; de Ruiter

& Hildebrand, 2003; see also Chapter 2 of this thesis). The average duration of residential treatment at the Dr. Henri van der Hoeven Kliniek is approximately four years.

## SUBJECTS

In total, the study sample consisted of a mixed sample of 107 patients (98 men, 9 women) with DSM Axis I and/or Axis II disorders, which can be considered representative for forensic psychiatric patients in the Netherlands. A subset of 60 patients (51 men, 9 women) took part in the study of the interrater reliability of the PCL-R. Participants in the study of the psychometric properties of the Dutch PCL-R (internal consistency, factor structure) were 98 male patients. Earlier findings (e.g., Strachan, Williamson, & Hare, 1990, cited in Hare, 1991; also Silverthorn & Frick, 1997) suggest that there may be sex differences in the behavioral manifestations of PCL-R psychopathy. To exclude possible confounding influences, we therefore chose to examine internal consistency and factor structure in male patients only. Table 1 presents demographic and diagnostic characteristics of the total sample.

Mean age upon admission to the hospital was 31.5 years ($SD$ = 8.0; range 19-50) for the total sample (men: $M$ = 31.3, $SD$ = 7.9; women: $M$ = 33.6, $SD$ = 9.3). In terms of ethnic origin, 77% of the sample was White, 14% was Afro-Caribbean, 6% was Mediterranean, and 4% other (e.g., Indonesian, Korean). Eighty-five patients (79%) were single. In terms of offenses, 52% of the sample was convicted for (attempted) murder/homicide, 23% for sexual offenses (e.g., rape, pedosexual offenses), 8% for robbery with violence, 7% for arson, and the rest for (aggravated) assault or extortion.

Based on all available data, consensus DSM-IV Axis I disorders were established for all patients by MH and CdR, in cooperation with a senior-diagnostician and a senior psychotherapist of the hospital staff. Forty-nine patients (46%) met criteria for at least one substance-related disorder (e.g., alcohol, cannabis, polysubstance abuse/dependence); 14 patients (13%) met criteria for schizophrenia or other psychotic disorders and 7 for mood disorders. In addition, 18 patients (17%) received a diagnosis of paraphilia.

The Dutch language version (Van den Brink & de Jong, 1992; De Jong, Derks, van Oel, & Rinne, 1997) of the Structured Interview for Personality Disorders (SIDP-R; Pfohl, Blum, Zimmerman, & Stangl, 1989; SIDP-IV; Pfohl, Blum, & Zimmerman, 1997) was used for the assessment of DSM-III-R/DSM-IV personality disorders (PDs).[2] The prevalence of PDs was substantial in this sample. Nineteen patients met criteria for paranoid PD, 8 for schizoid PD or schizotypal PD, 47 for antisocial PD, 29 for borderline PD, 7 for histrionic PD, 26 for narcissistic PD, 14 for avoidant PD, 6 for dependent PD, 11 for obsessive-compulsive PD and 5 for passive- aggressive PD. Co-morbidity on Axis II was more common than a single diagnosis. Of the 87 patients given a PD diagnosis, 56 (64%) received multiple diagnoses. The mean number of PDs per patient for patients with at least one diagnosis was 2.1.

TABLE 1
*Sample Characteristics (N = 107)*

|  | n | % |
|---|---|---|
| **Sex** |  |  |
| Male | 98 | 91.6 |
| Female | 9 | 8.4 |
| **Age (in years)** |  |  |
| 18-30 | 54 | 50.5 |
| 31-40 | 36 | 33.6 |
| 41-50 | 17 | 15.9 |
| **Ethnic origin** |  |  |
| White | 82 | 76.6 |
| Afro-Caribbean | 15 | 14.0 |
| Mediterranean | 6 | 5.6 |
| Other | 4 | 3.8 |
| **Index offense** |  |  |
| Murder/homicide | 56 | 52.3 |
| Sexual offense | 25 | 23.4 |
| Robbery | 8 | 7.5 |
| Arson | 7 | 6.5 |
| Other | 11 | 10.3 |

(*table continues*)

---

[2] Our initial use of DSM-III-R diagnoses was dictated by the duration of the data collection, which started before the SIDP-IV interview became available.

**TABLE 1** (*cont.*)

| | n | % |
|---|---|---|
| **Axis I diagnosis** | | |
| Any Axis I disorder | 91 | 85.0 |
| Any substance abuse/dependence | 49 | 45.8 |
| Psychotic disorder | 14 | 13.1 |
| Mood disorder | 7 | 6.5 |
| Paraphilia | 18 | 16.8 |
| Pathological gambling | 11 | 10.3 |
| **Axis II diagnosis** | | |
| Paranoid | 19 | 18.4 |
| Schizoid | 8 | 7.8 |
| Schizotypal | 8 | 7.8 |
| Antisocial | 47 | 45.6 |
| Borderline | 29 | 28.2 |
| Histrionic | 7 | 6.8 |
| Narcissistic | 26 | 25.2 |
| Avoidant | 14 | 13.6 |
| Dependent | 6 | 5.8 |
| Obsessive-compulsive | 11 | 10.7 |
| Passive-aggressive | 5 | 4.9 |
| Any Axis II disorder | 87 | 84.5 |

*Note.* DSM-III-R/DSM-IV Axis II diagnoses of 103 patients.

## ASSESSMENT

Since January 1996, newly admitted patients have been assessed upon admission (T1; baseline assessment) with a standardized psychological assessment battery. In order to provide information on treatment progress, all patients in our hospital are re-tested 18-24 months after admission (T2; follow-up 1), and again 42 months after admission (T3; follow-up 2). In November 1997, we also implemented PCL-R psychopathy assessment within our hospital.

PCL-R ratings of all patients in the study were based on the Dutch translation of the semi-structured interview schedule designed by Hare (1991) and a review of all the collateral information arriving with each patient upon admission to the hospital. The Hare PCL-R interview is a comprehensive interview concerning school adjustment, work history, future goals, finances, family background, sexual and intimate relationships, child and adolescent antisocial behavior and adult delinquency. For all patients, extensive collateral information was available, consisting of earlier psychiatric and psychological assessments for the court (at least one psychiatric and psychological evaluation per patient), police reports of past and current offense(s), prior commitments to treatment facilities, and information on family background. The authorized Dutch translation of the Hare PCL-R manual and the scoring sheet were used (Vertommen, Verheul, de Ruiter, & Hildebrand, 2002).

## RATERS AND TRAINING

In total, a pool of 10 raters (three men, seven women) was used to administer the PCL-R interviews. Four raters (the authors) took part in the interrater reliability study. Seven raters were M.A. (clinical) psychologists; two raters had a degree in mental health science (M.Sc.) of whom one (MH) also had a degree in law, and one rater is a Ph.D. clinical and forensic psychologist (CdR). All raters were familiar with DSM-IV Axis I/Axis II disorders (American Psychiatric Association, 1994) and had experience in psychological assessment and/or treatment of (forensic) psychiatric patients. All raters were trained extensively in administration and scoring of the PCL-R, either by Drs. Robert D. Hare and David Cooke in a three-day PCL-R workshop held at the Dr. Henri van der Hoeven Kliniek in October 1997; by Drs. Robert D. Hare and Stephen D. Hart in a three-day PCL-R workshop (Nijmegen, April 2000), or by Dr. Stephen D. Hart in a PCL-R workshop in Amsterdam (February 2001). In addition, the four raters who took part in the interrater reliability study (see Procedure) reviewed videotaped interviews of four patients and discussed PCL-R scores in detail to improve and sharpen the coding of the PCL-R criteria, prior to the reliability study.

## PROCEDURE

As a general rule, PCL-R interviews are videotaped in our hospital. However, patients have to give their written informed consent before videotaping the interview. Thus, patients were selected on their willingness to give informed consent and to cooperate with the interview process. If a patient refused to give informed consent for videotaping the interview, one rater conducted the interview while a second rater was present as an observer. After independent review of all available information (interview and file information), each rater scored the PCL-R and a meeting was planned to obtain a final (consensus) rating for that patient. This procedure, which is recommended by Hare (1991, 1998c), was chosen to maximize scoring accuracy. The PCL-R consensus scores are used in all subsequent data-analyses. If a patient refused videotaping the interview and also the presence of a second observer during the interview, PCL-R scores were based on the judgment of a single interviewer ($n = 7$). In all other cases, PCL-R consensus scores were based on independent PCL-R ratings of at least two independent raters.

To determine the interrater reliability of the PCL-R, videotaped interviews of 60 patients were rated independently by the interviewer and by two raters who watched the videotape of the interview (video versus vis-à-vis interview). In this way we were able to study the potential influence of information source on the PCL-R score (source effect). We do not know of any prior research that investigated the role of interview source in PCL-R ratings. Therefore, we could not draw on previous findings to set an expected effect size. However, because PCL-R ratings are only partially based on interview data, we expected the size of the source effect to be small. For analysis of variance with equal $Ns$ in three samples (i.e., videorater 1 versus videorater 2 versus interviewer) a small effect size, in terms of $f$, is "generally found in the .00 - .40 range" (Cohen, 1988, p. 284). The power value of the $F$ test for the main effect of source, given a significance level $\alpha$ of .05, effect size $f = .20$, sample size $n = 60$ and degrees of freedom for the numerator of the $F$ ratio = 2, is given as .67. This means that the a priori probability of rejecting the null hypothesis (i.e., the hypothesis that there is a source effect) is .67. For $\alpha = .05$ and $f = .40$, the power is .99.

The PCL-R interviews in the interrater reliability study were conducted by three of the four raters. PCL-R interviews with female patients ($n = 9$) were equally distributed among the interviewers. Each interviewer conducted 20 interviews and also rated 15 videotaped interviews from each of the other two interviewers. The fourth rater viewed 30 videotaped interviews conducted by the interviewers, 10 of each interviewer. All raters had access to the same collateral information. Occasionally, raters had been in contact with the patient previously for other psychodiagnostic activities (especially for patients interviewed at T2). However, none of the raters had been in contact previously with a patient for psychotherapy. The mean duration of the 60 PCL-R interviews in the reliability study was 165 minutes ($SD = 47$), varying from 50 to 296 minutes.

## RESULTS

### DESCRIPTIVE STATISTICS

The mean total consensus score of the PCL-R for the 98 male patients was 21.3 ($SD = 8.4$), with a range from 3 to 38, a median score of 21.1 and a mode of 17.0 (Table 2).

TABLE 2
*Descriptive Statistics, Internal Consistency (Cronbach's α), Item Homogeneinity (mean inter-item correlation), and Interrater Reliability (intraclass correlation coefficient; ICC) of PCL-R Total and Factor Scores*

|               | Mean | SD  | Internal consistency | Item homogeneity | Interrater reliability |
|---------------|------|-----|----------------------|------------------|------------------------|
| PCL-R total   | 21.3 | 8.4 | .87                  | .26              | .88                    |
| PCL-R Factor 1| 9.4  | 3.7 | .83                  | —                | .76                    |
| PCL-R Factor 2| 9.1  | 5.0 | .83                  | —                | .83                    |

*Note.* PCL-R = Psychopathy Checklist-Revised. PCL-R scores are adjusted sums of 98 male patients. For ICCs, $N = 60$. Single rater ICCs were calculated using a two-way random effects model. '—' = not calculated.

A *t*-test revealed no significant difference between the total PCL-R scores of White ($n = 75$) versus non-White ($n = 23$) participants, $t$ (96) = .21, n.s. The kurtosis of the PCL-R score was $-.77$ ($SE = .49$). PCL-R scores were normally distributed, Kolmogorov-Smirnov $Z = .60.$, $p = .86$. The mean Factor 1 score was 9.4 ($SD = 3.7$) and the mean Factor 2 score was 9.1 ($SD = 5.0$). For female patients ($n = 9$), the mean total score was

12.2 (*SD* = 6.7; range from 2 to 22), the mean Factor 1 score was 5.2 (*SD* = 3.0), and the mean Factor 2 score was 5.2 (*SD* = 3.2). When a cut-off point of 26 was applied, which is often used in European research (Grann, Långström, Tengström, & Stålenheim, 1998; Rasmussen, Storsæter, & Levander, 1999), 32 of the male patients (33%) were classified as 'psychopaths.'

It can be seen from Table 3 that individual PCL-R item means ranged between 0.36 for Item 17 (*Many short-term marital relationships*) to 1.55 for Item 16 (*Failure to accept responsibility for own actions*). Table 3 further indicates that a relatively high proportion of missing values was found for Items 17 (*Many short-term marital relationships*; 11%) and 19 (*Revocation of conditional release*; 28%).

## RELIABILITY ANALYSIS

*Interrater reliability.* Interrater reliability for PCL-R total and factor scores, as well as for individual PCL-R items was estimated by means of the intraclass correlation coefficient (ICC; Shrout & Fleiss, 1979; McGraw & Wong, 1996). This coefficient expresses the reliability of a rating by one rater generalized to the population of raters, from which the sample of raters was taken. In other words, ICCs estimate the equivalence of repeated measurements made on the same subjects. The following categories are often used for evaluating the observed reliability (Fleiss, 1986): $R \geq 0.75$ = excellent; $0.40 \leq R < 0.75$ = fair to good; $R < 0.40$ = poor. A two-way random effects model type was used for computing the ICC. With the use of a two-way ANOVA, it is possible to measure how much of the total variance in the observed scores is a result of between-subject variation, between-rater variation and uncontrollable (random) variation. The random effects model is appropriate when the raters involved in the study are a random sample of a population of possible raters who will later use the instrument under evaluation. Because raters were not crossed with patients in one $60 \times 3$ design, it is best to describe the interrater reliability study as consisting of one $30 \times 3$ design and three $10 \times 3$ designs. Given the unequal *n*s, weighted average single measure ICC correlations were calculated for individual PCL-R items, as well as for PCL-R Factor 1, Factor 2, and total scores.

The single measure ICC for the PCL-R total score was .88; for Factor 1, it was .76, and for Factor 2, it was .83. At the level of individual PCL-R items, in general, ICCs were good to excellent (*Mdn* = .67, range .46 to .80). Table 3 details interrater reliabilities for all PCL-R items. The highest single measure ICCs were obtained for Items 3 (*Need for stimulation/proneness to boredom*; .80), and 11 (*Promiscuous sexual behavior*; .80). Four items, including three loading on Factor 1, had reliabilities less than .60. Interrater reliabilities of PCL-R Factor 1 items tend to be slightly lower than reliabilities of Factor 2 items (*Mdn* ICC for Factor 1 = .63, for Factor 2 = .67).

Agreement on PCL-R categorical diagnoses was assessed using generalized Cohen's kappa (κ; Cohen, 1980). This statistic indicates the agreement between raters corrected for agreement by chance, and is considered the standard index of diagnostic agreement for categorical data (Shrout, Spitzer, & Fleiss, 1987). The same diagnostic categories that are used for evaluating the ICCs are used for evaluating the kappa. Comparison of PCL-R categorical diagnoses among the three raters showed good agreement, weighted average Cohens's κ = .72, for the presence versus absence of PCL-R psychopathy (adjusted sum total score ≥ 26). Furthermore, in 53 of the 60 cases (88%) the raters agreed on the presence or absence of psychopathy (PCL-R ≥ 26); 18 patients (30%) received a diagnosis of psychopathy from at least one of the three raters, 14 patients (23%) received a psychopathy diagnosis from at least two raters, while all three raters gave eight patients (13%) a psychopathy diagnosis. In addition, in 43 of the 60 cases (72%), PCL-R adjusted total scores between the three raters did not differ more than five points. In two cases, however, rather extreme differences (≥ 10 points) between raters were found.

**TABLE 3**
*Frequency of Item Scores, Descriptive Statistics, Corrected Item-Total Correlations, and Interrater Reliability (intraclass correlation coefficient; ICC) of Individual PCL-R Items*

| Item description | Value label 0 | 1 | 2 | — | Mean | SD | Item-total r | ICC |
|---|---|---|---|---|---|---|---|---|
| 1. Glibness/superficial charm | 58 | 24 | 16 | 0 | 0.57 | 0.76 | .49 | .46 |
| 2. Grandiose sense of self worth | 30 | 38 | 30 | 0 | 1.00 | 0.79 | .38 | .51 |
| 3. Needs stimulation/prone to boredom | 27 | 39 | 32 | 0 | 1.05 | 0.78 | .60 | .80 |
| 4. Pathological lying | 29 | 44 | 25 | 0 | 0.96 | 0.74 | .53 | .65 |
| 5. Conning/manipulative | 20 | 35 | 43 | 0 | 1.23 | 0.77 | .51 | .66 |
| 6. Lack of remorse or guilt | 10 | 35 | 53 | 0 | 1.44 | 0.67 | .63 | .69 |
| 7. Shallow affect | 13 | 49 | 36 | 0 | 1.23 | 0.67 | .26 | .60 |
| 8. Callous/lack of empathy | 13 | 49 | 36 | 0 | 1.23 | 0.67 | .45 | .52 |
| 9. Parasitic lifestyle | 39 | 32 | 24 | 3 | 0.84 | 0.80 | .64 | .68 |
| 10. Poor behavioral controls | 22 | 32 | 44 | 0 | 1.22 | 0.79 | .47 | .65 |
| 11. Promiscuous sexual behavior | 32 | 16 | 48 | 2 | 1.17 | 0.90 | .14 | .80 |
| 12. Early behavior problems | 63 | 17 | 15 | 3 | 0.49 | 0.76 | .33 | .79 |
| 13. Lack of realistic, long term goals | 37 | 24 | 37 | 0 | 1.00 | 0.87 | .59 | .52 |
| 14. Impulsivity | 22 | 37 | 39 | 0 | 1.17 | 0.77 | .57 | .67 |
| 15. Irresponsibility | 16 | 32 | 50 | 0 | 1.35 | 0.75 | .56 | .63 |
| 16. Failure to accept responsibility | 10 | 24 | 64 | 0 | 1.55 | 0.68 | .51 | .67 |
| 17. Many short-term marital relations | 66 | 11 | 10 | 11 | 0.36 | 0.68 | .40 | .79 |
| 18. Juvenile delinquency | 47 | 16 | 31 | 4 | 0.83 | 0.90 | .36 | .78 |
| 19. Revocation of conditional release | 17 | 9 | 45 | 27 | 1.39 | 0.85 | .42 | .77 |
| 20. Criminal versatility | 26 | 30 | 42 | 0 | 1.16 | 0.82 | .60 | .76 |

*Note.* PCL-R = Psychopathy Checklist-Revised. '—' = number of omitted items. Item frequencies, means and standard deviations, and item-total correlations are based on PCL-R consensus ratings from 98 male patients. For interrater reliability analyses, $N = 60$. Due to omitted items by at least one of the raters, ICCs for item 4 ($n = 59$), item 9 ($n = 59$), item 12 ($n = 57$), item 17 ($n = 54$), item 18 ($n = 57$), and item 19 ($n = 38$) are based on smaller sample sizes. Single rater ICCs were calculated using a two-way random effects model. All ICCs were significantly greater than 0 ($p < .05$).

*Interviewer ratings versus ratings conducted by video-observers.* A source (interview versus video) by rater (Raters 1 through 4) ANOVA was performed on all individual PCL-R items and the PCL-R total score. Neither the main effects for source and rater, nor the Source × Rater interaction, were significant for any of the PCL-R items or the

PCL-R total score. This indicates that the information source (i.e., real-life interview versus a videotaped interview) did not affect the scoring of the rater to a significant degree.

*Internal consistency.* The internal consistency of the PCL-R was examined in the sample of 98 male patients using Cronbach's coefficient alpha, and was found to be high, alpha = .87, with an alpha coefficient of .83 obtained for Factors 1 and 2. These figures are comparable to those obtained with the standardization sample (Hare, 1991). To provide a more fine-grained analysis of internal consistency, we also examined corrected item-total correlations for each PCL-R item in this sample (see Table 3). With the exception of Items 7 (*Shallow affect*), 11 (*Promiscuous sexual behavior*), and 12 (*Early behavior problems*), all items had corrected item-to-total correlations ≥ .35, indicating that they all contribute significantly to the PCL-R total score; 10 of the 20 items had item-total correlations of .50 or higher. The highest correlations were obtained for Items 9 (*Parasitic lifestyle*; $r$ = .64) and 6 (*Lack of remorse or guilt*; $r$ = .63). The mean inter-item correlation[3] was .26, which is above the suggested cut-off of .20 for a scale to be considered homogeneous (Green, Lissitz, & Mulaik, 1977).

## FACTOR ANALYSIS

To determine whether the oblique two-factor structure of the PCL-R (Hare, 1991; Harpur et al., 1989) could be replicated in the current sample of 98 male forensic psychiatric patients, a confirmatory factor analysis (CFA) was performed. The question in CFA is whether the correlations among variables are consistent with a hypothesized factor structure. Compared to exploratory FA, CFA offers more definitive empirical evidence of the underlying factor structure of a scale (Floyd & Widaman, 1995). Model feasibility was assessed using LISREL 8 (Jöreskog & Sörbom, 1993), with maximum likelihood estimation. A simple factor structure was modeled with eight variables loading on Factor 1 and nine variables loading on Factor 2 as in the original solution (Hare, 1991; Harpur et al., 1989). Because each measure of fit has limitations and no agreed methods for absolutely

---

[3] Following Hare (1991), we carried out different analyses to determine the most appropriate method for assigning a value to a missing item (e.g., scoring a missing value using the mean score for that item obtained in the sample, scoring a missing value as 1). Because it made little difference which method was used, we decided to use the simplest method (assigning the value 1).

determining goodness of fit exist (Kline, 1998; Tabachnick & Fidell, 2001) the quality of fit was estimated using multiple indices.

Findings indicate that the two-factor model proposed by Hare (1991) did not fit our data well, $\chi^2$ (118, $N = 98$) = 561.8, $p < .001$, root mean square error of approximation (RMSEA) = .16 (90% CI = .14 - .17), standardized root mean square residual (SRMR) = .13, non-normed fit index (NNFI) = .50, comparative fit index (CFI) = .57. The estimates for those parameters between the items and the factors they were supposed to load on, ranged from 0.55 to 0.87, while the estimate for the covariance relationship between the two factors was 0.50. Post hoc model modifications were performed in an attempt to develop a better fitting model. On the basis of the Lagrange multiplier test, a path predicting Item 14 (*Impulsivity*) from Factor 1 (i.e., allowing Item 14 to load on Factor 2 as well as on Factor 1) was added. A chi-square difference test indicated that the model was significantly improved by addition of this path, change in $\chi^2$ (1, $N = 98$) = 20.9, $p < .001$. The modified model also indicated a bad fit, $\chi^2$ (117, $N = 98$) = 540.9, $p < .001$, RMSEA = .15 (90% CI = .14 - .17), SRMR = .12, NNFI = 52, CFI = .59. Examination of the modification indices suggested that allowing several errors of measurement to correlate would substantially improve the fit of the modified model. To this end, six errors of measurement were allowed to correlate.[4] Although the fit of this revised model was significantly improved, change in $\chi^2$ (6, $N = 98$) = 102.7, $p < .001$, the model still did not fit the data, $\chi^2$ (111, $N = 98$) = 438.2, $p < .001$, RMSEA = .13 (90% CI = .11 - .15), SRMR = .11, NNFI = 61, CFI = .68.

As the two-factor model did not appear to fit our data, the 13-item model developed by Cooke and Michie (2001) was used in a CFA. A factor structure was modeled with four items loading on the Arrogant and deceitful interpersonal style factor, four items on the factor Deficient affective experience, and five items on the Impulsive and irresponsible behavioral style factor. Examination of the fit statistics revealed that the three-factor model provided a poor fit to the data, $\chi^2$ (62, $N = 98$) = 433, $p < .001$, RMSEA = .21 (90% CI = .19 - .23), SRMR = .13, NNFI = .53, CFI = .62. Adding additional paths did not

---

[4] We choose the errors of measurement which were allowed to correlate on the basis of which items shared content beyond that related to the underlying construct: Items 1-2, 2-15, 6-16, 10-14, 12-18.

significantly improve the model. Also, allowing several errors of measurement to correlate did not result in a good fit of the model to the data.

Given the poor fit of our data to both the two-factor solution of Hare (1991) and the three-factor model developed by Cooke and Michie (2001) using CFA, we decided to investigate the factor structure of the Dutch language version of the PCL-R in the present sample by means of an exploratory principal components analysis (PCA). This analyses would also allow us to compare findings with other European research that examined the PCL-R factor structure with PCA (e.g., Hobson & Shine, 1998; Moltó et al., 2000). Analyses were conducted using SPSS 10.0 for Windows. The analysis revealed six components (factors) with eigenvalues greater than one, accounting for 68% of the total variance. The first two components accounted for 44% of the total variance. Visual inspection of the scree plot (Cattell, 1966) revealed a noticeable eigenvalue drop and leveling off after the second component. The unrotated first PC accounted for 30% of the variance in the PCL-R. The unrotated second PC accounted for 14% of the variance. The remaining factors accounted for 7%, 6%, 6%, and 5% of the variance, respectively, suggesting that a two-factor solution is sufficient for the data of this sample.

We assessed the relative suitability of a two-factor solution using PC extraction and oblimin rotation to account for the fact that the factors produced by the PC analysis were correlated. The results obtained showed a correlation of .25 between the two factors. Table 4 presents the two-factor solution for the present study. Variables are ordered and grouped by size of loadings to facilitate interpretation. Factor 1 consisted of nine items with loadings of .40 or above. The highest loadings were found for Items 14 (*Impulsivity*; .84), 20 (*Criminal versatility*; .78), 3 (*Need for stimulation/proneness to boredom*; .72), 10 (*Poor behavioral controls*; .68), and 15 (*Irresponsibility*; .68). Factor 2 also consisted of nine items with loadings of .4 or above. The highest loadings were found for Items 7 (*Shallow affect*; .71), 8 (*Callous/lack of empathy*; .70), 2 (*Grandiose sense of self worth*, .69), 1 (*Glibness/superficial charm*; .69), and 5 (*Conning/manipulative*; .66). The Items 11 (*Promiscuous sexual behavior*) and 17 (*Many short-term marital relationships*) did not load on either factor.

TABLE 4

*Psychopathy Checklist-Revised Two Factor Oblique Solution (Delta = 0; pattern matrix) for a Sample of 98 Male Forensic Psychiatric Patients*

| | | PCL-R | |
|---|---|---|---|
| **Item number and description** | | Factor 1 | Factor 2 |
| 14. Impulsivity | (2) | **84** | -09 |
| 20. Criminal versatility | — | **78** | 02 |
| 3. Need for stimulation/prone to boredom | (2) | **72** | 09 |
| 10. Poor behavioral controls | (2) | **68** | -04 |
| 15. Irresponsibility | (2) | **68** | 09 |
| 12. Early behavior problems | (2) | **63** | -17 |
| 18. Juvenile delinquency | (2) | **58** | -06 |
| 9. Parasitic lifestyle | (2) | **54** | 37 |
| 19. Revocation of conditional release | (2) | **52** | -08 |
| 7. Shallow affect | (1) | -25 | **71** |
| 8. Callous/lack of empathy | (1) | -02 | **70** |
| 2. Grandiose sense of self worth | (1) | -09 | **69** |
| 1. Glibness/superficial charm | (1) | 01 | **69** |
| 5. Conning/manipulative | (1) | 10 | **66** |
| 6. Lack of remorse or guilt | (1) | 31 | **58** |
| 4. Pathological lying | (1) | 21 | **58** |
| 16. Failure to accept responsibility | (1) | 24 | **52** |
| 13. Lack of realistic, long-term goals | (2) | 38 | **46** |
| 17. Many short-term marital relationships | — | 35 | 17 |
| 11. Promiscuous sexual behavior | — | -06 | 32 |
| Initial eigen values | | 6.0 | 2.7 |
| Percentage of variance | | 30.1 | 13.6 |

*Note.* This solution was obtained by specifying a two-factor solution. Decimal points are omitted and loadings > 0.4 are in bold; factor denotation from Hare's factor solution as described in the PCL-R manual are in parentheses. A '—' indicates that the item does not load on either factor.

## DISCUSSION

The present findings provide initial evidence for the interrater reliability of the Dutch version of the PCL-R. In a sample of 60 forensic psychiatric patients, interrater reliabilities of the individual PCL-R items were demonstrated to be good to excellent. The single measure ICC for the PCL-R total score was .88; for Factor 1, it was .76, and for Factor 2, it was .83. The high levels of reliability found in the present study are consistent with those documented by other researchers. Indeed, cross-cultural research (e.g., Cooke, 1996, 1998; Moltó et al., 2000) supports the reliability of the Hare PCL-R. The reliabilities of the PCL-R items reported in many studies are generally high, although reliability coefficients vary per item, in part depending on the ease with which particular PCL-R items can be rated (Cooke, 1998). Hare et al. (1990) assessed interrater reliability using either a joint interview approach or the second rater observed a videotape of the interview in a large sample of prisoners and forensic psychiatric patients. For subsamples of subjects, ICC coefficients for the PCL-R total score ranged from .78 to .94 ($M = .86$) for a single rating. In addition, Moltó et al. (2000), using a joint interview approach to assess interrater reliability of the PCL-R in 49 adult male Spanish prisoners, reported ICC coefficients ranging from .87 to .96 for a single rating using a one-way random effects model. Note that we had the disposal of *three* independent PCL-R ratings per patient, which is an extremely thorough examination of interrater reliability, far more thorough than, for example, the often practiced joint-interview approach (Zimmerman, 1994). The categorical diagnosis of PCL-R psychopathy was also reliable (weighted average $\kappa = .72$, for simultaneous comparison of three raters). There were considerable differences between the raters with regard to clinical experience, training and background, but this did not result in significant differences in diagnostic reliability, demonstrated by the fact that there was no rater effect.

The Dutch language PCL-R has excellent internal consistency (Cronbach's $\alpha = .88$ for the PCL-R total score). This figure is comparable to those obtained in the standardization samples (Hare, 1991). Also, we found adequate item-total correlations. Except for Items 6 (*Lack of remorse or guilt*), 11 (*Promiscuous sexual behavior*), and 12 (*Early behavioral problems*), the corrected item-total correlations were $\geq .35$, indicating they all contributed significantly to the PCL-R total score. Both internal consistency and item-total correlations were quite similar to the findings reported by other scholars, for instance, Hare et al. (1990; Cronbach's $\alpha = .88$; mean inter-item correlation = .27) and Moltó et al. (2000; Cronbach's $\alpha = .85$; mean inter-item correlation = .22).

With regard to a possible source effect (interview versus video) in rating the PCL-R, it was hypothesized that (particularly) PCL-R Factor 1 items would be susceptible to such an effect. However, we did not find a significant effect of information source on ratings of individual PCL-R items or the total score. We believe that the absence of a difference between interviewer and videotape ratings is most likely due to the fact that the information required to score the PCL-R depends as much on the extensive collateral information available as on the information provided by the interview. It may be that impressions based on real-life interviews do in fact differ from those based on videotaped interviews, because the latter do not include face-to-face interaction. These impressions may influence judgments, particularly on the "soft" Factor 1 items of the PCL-R (Cooke, 1995, p.111). Thus, variability between raters in their impressions is a possible source of difference, and may negatively affect interrater reliability. Indeed, ICCs of PCL-R Factor 1 items were the lowest of the individual PCL-R items, especially in comparison to several behavioral items (e.g., early behavior problem, juvenile delinquency, criminal versatility). However, many PCL-R items are largely scored on the basis of collateral information (psychiatric or psychological evaluations, and police files), which might 'overrule' the impressions gathered from the interview (either interview or video). This might explain the large overall degree of convergence between video and interviewer ratings, especially because the available file information was quite extensive in this study. Our findings corroborate those of Grann, Långström, Tengström, and Stålenheim (1998), who demonstrated good reliability between independent clinical PCL-R ratings (based on interview and file information) and retrospective file-only ratings, in part because the files were of good quality.

The finding that the PCL-R can be scored reliably from a videotaped interview (in combination with collateral information) has some practical implications. If, due to limited resources in a particular (forensic) setting, it is not possible to get two independent PCL-R ratings, a trained rater from a different facility could score the PCL-R on the basis of a videotaped interview, in order to provide the necessary second rating. Furthermore, videotaped interviews could be used in court cases, for example when a second opinion is asked for.

Confirmatory factor analysis showed that both Hare's two-factor model and the three-factor model identified by Cooke and Michie (2001) did not fit our data. Although this study was not intended as a model modification study, we conducted supplementary analyses in an attempt to develop a better fitting model. However, allowing items to load on more than one factor or allowing a number of errors of measurement to correlate did not significantly improve the fit of the models tested. It should be noted that it is difficult to obtain acceptable confirmatory solutions in cases of violation of assumptions, such as small sample size and noninterval scaling of items (e.g., Floyd & Widaman, 1995). Our sample was relatively small, although there is no generally accepted guideline for sample size in case of CFA (Floyd & Widaman, 1995; see also below). Ideally, CFA is performed on interval or quasi-interval scales, for instance 5- or 7-point Likert scales; the PCL-R's 3-point scale does not meet this ideal.

The subsequent exploratory factor analysis yielded an oblique two-factor structure, accounting for 44% of the variance. Our first factor appeared to be similar to Hare's Factor 2. However, some notable differences were found. First, Item 20 (*Criminal versatility*) loaded high on our first factor but did not load on Hare's Factor 2. Second, Item 13 (*Lack of realistic, long-term plans*) did not load on the antisocial lifestyle factor in the present study. Our second factor included the eight items of Hare's Factor 1 plus Item 13 (*Lack of realistic long-term goals*). The Items 11 (*Promiscuous sexual behavior*) and 17 (*Many short-term marital relationships*) did not to load on either factor, as was the case in Hare's two-factor model.

Even though the use of confirmatory factor analytic techniques did not result in a replication of Hare's original two-factor model, our exploratory factor analysis pointed — at least to a certain extent — to a resemblance between our two-factor solution and Hare's. Several European scholars, employing exclusively exploratory factor analytic techniques, have claimed to find support for Hare's two-factor solution in their data, although some notable differences with the Hare solution exist. Hobson and Shine (1998), for example, examined the PCL-R factor structure in a sample of 104 inmates admitted to Grendon therapeutic prison. Similar to the present findings, and in contrast with Hare's two-factor solution, they found that Item 20 (*Criminal versatility*) loaded high on the antisocial lifestyle factor. Another difference was that Item 11 (*Promiscuous sexual behavior*) loaded on Factor 1 (*Selfish, callous and remorseless use of others*), while this item is not included in the Hare model. Likewise, Moltó et al. (2000), in a sample of 117 Spanish male prison inmates, found that Item 11 loaded significantly on (Hare's) Factor 1. The picture that emerges from these three European studies is that each study on it's own did not provide unequivocal support for Hare's two-factor model. Pooling of these and other European data, to increase sample size, would seem worthwhile, to further examine such fundamental questions as: (1) Which model (the two-factor or the three-factor model) fits the European PCL-R data better, and (2) What is the role of cultural differences (cf. Cooke, 1996, 1998; Cooke & Michie, 2001) in the expression of psychopathic traits? Recently, Skeem, Mulvey, and Grisso (2003) independently cross-validated the three-factor model of Cooke and Michie (2001) in a large sample ($N$ = 870) of civil psychiatric patients, using the Screening Version of the PCL. They concluded that "Cooke and Michie's (2001) three-factor model of psychopathy is more plausible than the traditional PCL two-factor model with these patients because it better describes the structure of the PCL:SV and more specifically assesses personality deviation" (p. 51). Using these recently-developed factorial approaches may yield important information about the robustness of these factors in diverse populations.

With regard to ethnic group differences in PCL-R scores, the present study found no difference between White and other subjects. Kosson et al. (1990), using a sample of Black and White inmates, found some race-related differences in PCL-R scores. As Brandt et al. (1997) noted correctly, these differences were quite selective and have not been observed in other studies. Also, Cooke et al. (2001), using IRT methods to analyse PCL-R ratings of Caucasian and African-American adult male offenders, found no evidence of racial differences.

A few methodological limitations of the present study should be mentioned. First, interrater reliability data were available for 60 patients, which may be a relatively small sample size. A larger sample might have increased variability and therefore reliability estimates. At the very least, a larger sample would have resulted in more stable estimates. Second, one may argue that the high levels of interrater reliability found are due to a possible training effect caused by the PCL-R consensus meetings held after the three raters had independently scored the PCL-R for a particular patient. If this were the case, one would expect less divergence (higher levels of reliability) in the second half than in the first half of the series of 60 cases. However, single measure ICC values for the adjusted sum PCL-R total score were .89 for the first 20 of the 60 PCL-R ratings and .90 for the last

20 of the series. A *Z* test indicated that there was no significant difference between these correlations. Thus, there is no indication for a training effect.

A further limitation includes the small sample size for the study of the factor structure of the PCL-R in relation to the number of variables. However, guidelines for sample size have always been varying, the general rule of thumb being "the more subjects, the better" (Floyd & Widaman, 1995, p. 289). Streiner (1994), for example, recommends adequate solutions would be obtained with five subjects per variable as long as there were about 100 subjects in the sample. Tabachnick and Fidell (2001) suggest using at least 300 cases for factor analysis, which can be problematic in practice. In our hospital, for example, it would take about 10 to 12 years to get 300 newly admitted patients.

To summarize, it can be concluded that the Dutch language version of the PCL-R is a reliable instrument for use with forensic psychiatric patients and that the PCL-R can be applied in the forensic psychiatric population in the Netherlands. The current study did not confirm Hare's two-factor structure nor the three-factor model identified by Cooke and Michie (2001). Exploratory principal components analysis using oblique rotation, however, identified two main factors which were, to a certain extent, comparable to those obtained by Hare (1991) in the standardization samples and in other Western European samples. As the use of the PCL-R is likely to increase in Dutch forensic psychiatric hospitals in the future, there is a need for normative Dutch data and validity research. More research with different, larger samples (e.g., female forensic psychiatric patients, prisoners) is needed to further support the scientific status of the instrument for the Dutch forensic field.

Chapter 4

# PREVALENCE OF PSYCHOPATHY
# AND ITS RELATION TO
# DSM-IV AXIS I AND AXIS II DISORDERS[1]

[1] Published as:
Hildebrand, M., & Ruiter, C. de. PCL-R psychopathy and its relation to DSM-IV Axis I and Axis II disorders in a sample of male Dutch forensic psychiatric patients. *International Journal of Law and Psychiatry, 27*, 233-248.
The authors are grateful to Cécile Vandeputte-van de Vijver and Daan van Beek, who aided in establishing DSM-IV Axis I diagnoses. We also would like to thank Robert D. Hare for his helpful comments.

## SUMMARY

The association between psychopathy and the DSM-IV classification of mental disorders (American Psychiatric Association, 1994) was examined in a sample of 98 male Dutch criminal offenders involuntarily admitted to a forensic psychiatric hospital. Psychopathy was assessed with Hare's Psychopathy Checklist-Revised (PCL-R). Axis I diagnoses were lifetime clinical diagnoses based on consensus between four independent raters. The Structured Interview for DSM-IV Disorders of Personality (SIDP-IV) was used for the assessment of Axis II disorders. The overall psychiatric morbidity in the sample was high. Co-morbidity was the rule, regardless of the degree of PCL-R psychopathy. Psychopathy was significantly positively related to non-alcohol substance use disorders, antisocial and Cluster B personality disorder (PD). Most patients with a PCL-R score $\geq 26$ had a DSM-IV antisocial PD; the reverse was not true. PCL-R scores were also positively correlated ($r \geq .33$) with dimensional scores of paranoid, borderline, and narcissistic PD, and with conduct disorder ($< 15$ years) and antisocial behavior since age 15.

# INTRODUCTION

Psychopathy was the first personality disorder to be recognized in psychiatry. According to Schneider (1923), a German psychiatrist, the term psychopathy referred to a variety of personality disorders (psychopathic personalities) as extreme variants of normal personality. It has been given many different labels (Hare, 1991), such as psychopathic inferiority, character deficiency, moral insanity, and manipulative personality. The current interest in the disorder is (at least partly) attributable to the development of the Hare Psychopathy Checklist-Revised (PCL-R) (Hare, 1991; Hare, Harpur et al., 1990) and the abundance of empirical research it has generated over the past two decades. PCL-R items are personality traits and behaviors, which are scored on a 3-point scale (2 = *the item definitely applies to the subject*, 1 = *the item applies to a certain extent*, 0 = *the item does not apply to the subject*), yielding a maximum total of 40. A score of 30 or more is recommended by Hare (1991) to identify the prototypical psychopath. PCL-R items define two correlated, oblique factors, Factor 1 (callous and remorseless style of relating to other people) primarily at high levels of the construct and Factor 2 (unstable, socially deviant lifestyle) at low levels of the construct (Cooke & Michie, 1997). Recently, however, Cooke and Michie (2001) using confirmatory factor analysis, identified distinct interpersonal, affective, and behavioral factors of which the measurement is uncontaminated by items reflecting antisocial behavior.

Evidence gathered in the last decade demonstrates that the PCL-R scale is highly reliable when used with trained and experienced raters. Studies in a variety of countries have typically obtained intraclass correlations (ICCs) > .80 for a single rater. Internal consistency (alpha coefficients > .80; mean inter-item correlations > .22) is also high. Considerable evidence has accrued attesting to the construct-related validity of the PCL-R. In several (mostly North American) studies (Hart & Hare, 1989; Hemphill, Hart, & Hare, 1994; Schroeder, Schroeder, & Hare, 1983; Smith & Newman, 1990) an expected pattern of relations with clinical assessments of DSM-III(-R) Axis I and Axis II disorders (American Psychiatric Association, 1980, 1987) is reported, the interpretation of which is greatly clarified by analysis of the two-factor structure of the PCL-R (Hart & Hare, 1997). In addition, there is increasing evidence that PCL-R scores are related, in appropriate ways, to so-called psychopathy-related self-report scales, as well as to a wide variety of behavioral variables (Bodholt, Richards, & Gacono, 2000; Hare, 1991; Hart & Hare, 1997).

The most common finding in studies that have examined the association between PCL-R psychopathy and DSM-III(-R) Axis I mental disorders, is that a diagnosis of PCL-R psychopathy is rarely significantly associated with individual Axis I pathology other than substance use disorders (Blackburn, 1998a; Hart & Hare, 1989; Nedopil, Hollweg, Hartmann, & Jasper, 1998; Rice & Harris, 1995b; Stålenheim & von Knorring, 1996). Hart and Hare (1989), for example, reported that patients with a diagnosis of PCL-R psychopathy (total score ≥ 30) were nine times less likely to receive any Axis I principal diagnosis than were other patients. However, moderate to strong associations between the PCL-R total and Factor 2 scores and substance-related disorders, and weak relationships between Factor 1 scores and substance abuse were found (Hart & Hare, 1989; Rutherford, Alterman, & Cacciola, 2000). Smith and Newman (1990) assessed substance use disorder with a structured interview in 360 male prison inmates. Analyses revealed that PCL-R psychopathy was significantly associated with both alcohol and drug abuse/dependence disorders. Other studies (Hart, Hare, & Harpur, 1992; Hemphill, Hart et al., 1994) also found significant correlations between PCL/PCL-R scores and drug abuse/dependence diagnoses; however, correlations with alcohol abuse/dependence diagnoses were not significant. Similar associations were found in European samples of prisoners and forensic psychiatric patients (Andersen, Sestoft, Lillebæk, Mortensen, & Kramp, 1999; Stålenheim & von Knorring, 1996).

With regard to the association with personality disorders (PDs), the majority of PCL-R psychopaths meet the criteria for antisocial PD, whereas a large proportion of subjects with the antisocial PD diagnosis do not meet the PCL-R criteria for psychopathy (Blackburn, 1998a; Hart & Hare, 1989; Stålenheim & von Knorring, 1996). The correlation between PCL-R scores and (dimensional) diagnoses of antisocial PD is usually quite high, i.e., $r = .55$ to $.65$ (Hart & Hare, 1989). The prevalence rates of (PCL-R) psychopathy among samples of forensic subjects (15 - 30%), however, are much lower than those for the DSM diagnosis of antisocial PD (50 - 80%) (Hare, 1985; Hart, Hare, & Forth, 1994). Results further indicate that the PCL-R score correlates positively with DSM-

III(-R) Axis II Cluster B disorders ("dramatic-erratic-emotional") and negatively with Cluster C personality, the "anxious-fearful" cluster (Hart & Hare, 1985; Hart, Hare, & Forth, 1994). Rutherford, Alterman, Cacciola, and McKay (1997), for example, found strong and significant correlations between the PCL-R total score and the number of symptoms of DSM-III-R APD, borderline, narcissistic, and histrionic PD in a sample of 250 male methadone patients. Hart and Hare (1989) reported positive correlations between PCL-R total scores and categorical diagnoses of DSM-III antisocial and histrionic PD in a sample of 80 North American men remanded by the courts for inpatient assessment of competency to stand trial. PCL-R Factor 1 scores were negatively correlated with prototypicality ratings of avoidant and dependent PD. A diagnosis of psychopathy was significantly associated with only one DSM-III Axis II disorder, namely APD (odds ratio = 11.32). Finally, examining 61 Swedish male forensic psychiatric patients, Stålenheim and von Knorring (1996) found that PCL-R defined psychopathy was strongly associated with the presence of Cluster B disorders ($t = 7.89$, $p < .0001$) and a diagnosis of antisocial personality disorder ($\chi^2 = 27.9$, $p < .001$) according to DSM-III-R criteria.

To summarize, previous work has generally supported the construct validity of Hare's PCL-R in relation to assessments of DSM-III(-R) Axis I and Axis II disorders, based on semi-structured interviews. Most of this work, however, has involved North American criminal and forensic samples. We do not know whether the findings reported are generalizable to European forensic psychiatric samples. In addition, to the best of our knowledge, no study has been published that systematically examined the association between PCL-R psychopathy and *DSM-IV* Axis I and Axis II disorders (American Psychiatric Association, 1994).

## AIM OF THE STUDY

The current study was designed to examine the association between PCL-R scores and (a) assessments of DSM-IV Axis I disorders and (b) diagnoses of DSM-III-R/DSM-IV Axis II disorders made on the basis of a semi-structured interview, the preferred method of assessment in personality disorder research (Loranger, 1992; Zimmerman, 1994), in a sample of forensic psychiatric patients. On the basis of earlier findings we expected PCL-R scores to be negatively correlated with individual Axis I disorders, except for substance use disorders, and to be positively associated with personality disorders of the "dramatic-erratic-emotional" cluster and negatively with personality disorders of the "anxious-fearful" cluster.

## METHOD

### SETTING

The study was conducted in the Dr. Henri van der Hoeven Kliniek, a Dutch forensic psychiatric facility for the residential treatment of criminal offenders who are sentenced by the court to involuntary commitment because of diminished responsibility for the crimes they committed. In terms of legal status, patients are sentenced by the court to a *maatregel van terbeschikkingstelling* (TBS-order). The purpose of the Dutch TBS-order is to protect society from unacceptably high risks of recidivism, through involuntary admission to a forensic psychiatric hospital, and through the treatment provided there (de Ruiter & Hildebrand, 2003). Every one or two years the court re-evaluates the patient in order to determine whether the risk of recidivism is still too high and treatment needs to be continued. Most patients serve a limited prison sentence before they are hospitalized.

### SUBJECTS

Subjects were 98 male forensic psychiatric patients admitted to the hospital between January 1, 1996 and December 1, 2001 with whom we were able to administer the PCL-R: (a) based on the results of an interview and (b) extensive collateral information. The sample represents approximately 75% of available male subjects admitted to the hospital between January 1, 1996 and December 1, 2001. The remainder were either not examined or provided incomplete data as a result of refusal of an interview, referral to another facility, or their clinical symptoms.

The mean age at admission was 31.5 years (*SD* = 7.8; range = 19 - 50). Most (78%) of the patients were White, and the rest were Surinamese/Antillian (13%), Mediterranean (7%) or other descent. Sixty-six patients (67%) had never been married nor lived in a common law marriage. Fifty percent of the sample was convicted for (attempted) murder/homicide, and 25% for sexual offences (e.g., sexual assault, rape, child molest); the others for (aggravated) assault, robbery with violence, threat, and arson.

## ASSESSMENTS

*Psychopathy.* Psychopathy was assessed with the PCL-R, following the guidelines provided by Hare (1991). PCL-R assessments of all patients were based on the results of an interview with the patient on the basis of the Dutch language version of the semi-structured PCL-R interview designed by Hare (1991). Also, for all patients, file records consisting of elaborate psychiatric and psychological evaluations, police records, criminal history, and family background data were reviewed. The authorized Dutch translation of the Hare PCL-R manual was used (Vertommen, Verheul, de Ruiter, & Hildebrand, 2002). Items were summed to yield three scores: Factor 1 ('callous and remorseless use of others'), Factor 2 ('chronically unstable and antisocial lifestyle') and the PCL-R total score (Hare, 1991). In the present study the item scoring for the two factors derived by Hare, Harpur et al. (1990) was used.

PCL-R interviews are generally videotaped, for which patients have to give their written informed consent. Thus, patients were selected on their willingness to give informed consent and to cooperate with the interview process. As a general procedure, PCL-R ratings were made by (at least) two independent raters. Nineteen patients refused to give consent for videotaping the interview; 13 of them agreed with a joint interview approach (one rater conducted the interview while a second rater was present as an observer); 6 refused the presence of a second observer, and PCL-R scores had to be based on the judgment of a single interviewer (MH or CdR). In all other cases ($n = 92$), PCL-R scores were based on PCL-R ratings of at least two independent raters. Previously, we reported that comparisons between real-life interview and videotaped interview indicated that the information source (interview versus video) did not influence the raters' coding (Hildebrand, de Ruiter, de Vogel, & van der Wolf, 2002). After independent review of all available information (interview and file information), each rater scored the PCL-R and a meeting was planned to obtain a final (consensus) rating for each patient. This procedure, recommended by Hare (1991, 1998c) was chosen to optimize scoring accuracy. PCL-R consensus scores were used in all subsequent data-analyses. It should be noted that PCL-R scores for every patient were established by at least one rater who previously participated in the interrater reliability study of the Dutch language version of the PCL-R (Hildebrand et al., 2002). The interrater reliability appeared to be excellent. The intraclass correlation coefficient (ICC), using a two-way random effects model, for the PCL-R total score was .88 for a single rater (Factor 1 = .76; Factor 2 = .83). Ratings were also internally consistent (Cronbach's alpha for the PCL-R total score = .87). All raters had been trained in scoring the PCL-R either by Drs. Robert D. Hare and David Cooke in a three-day PCL-R basic and advanced workshop; by Drs. Robert D. Hare and Stephen D. Hart in a three day PCL-R workshop, or by Dr. Stephen D. Hart (see Chapter 3).

*DSM-IV Axis I disorders.* Consistent with earlier research (e.g., Coid, 1992; Rasmussen, Storsæter, & Levander, 1999; Timmerman & Emmelkamp, 2001), lifetime Axis I diagnoses were established by the first author (MH) using all available data (e.g., earlier psychological and psychiatric reports, earlier diagnoses, current psychiatric or psychological assessments). In order to be able to compare with other studies examining the prevalence of Axis I diagnoses, These diagnoses were reviewed by three independent raters: a senior-diagnostician and a senior psychotherapist of the hospital staff, and the second author. Missing diagnoses were added and disagreements between the four raters were discussed and resolved, and a set of final consensus diagnoses for all patients in the sample was established. This procedure (i.e., using consensus diagnoses) was chosen to maximize scoring accuracy. Diagnoses were clustered into the following categories: (a) organic disorders, (b) schizophrenia or other psychotic disorders, (c) mood disorders, (d) anxiety disorders, and (e) sexual disorders (paraphilia). In addition, the substance use diagnoses (i.e., abuse and dependence) were divided into two main categories: alcohol related disorders and other substance abuse/dependence (such as cannabis, polysubstance, sedative, and cocaine abuse/dependence). No interrater reliability data were collected for Axis I disorders.

*Axis II disorders.* PD diagnoses were obtained by administration of the Structured Interview for DSM-III-R (SIDP-R) (van den Brink & de Jong, 1992; Pfohl, Blum, Zimmerman, & Stangl, 1989;) or DSM-IV Disorders of Personality (SIDP-IV) (de Jong, Derks, van Oel, & Rinne, 1996; Pfohl, Blum, & Zimmerman, 1994). Our use of the SIDP-R is a consequence of the duration of the data collection, which started before the SIDP-IV became available. Eleven patients were diagnosed using the SIDP-R; the rest was diagnosed using the SIDP-IV.[2] The SIDP-R is a semi-structured interview consisting of 160 items designed to assess the criteria of the DSM-III-R PD's. Questions are grouped into 17 topical sections (not into PDs) such as interpersonal functioning, emotional expression, and perception of threat. The SIDP-IV assesses all DSM-IV PD's plus self-defeating PD of the DSM-III-R (sadistic PD is not included). The questions of the SIDP-IV are grouped into 10 topic areas, such as interests, emotions, and activities. Interviewers are free to make additional inquiries when necessary. The interviewers did not rate items while interviewing but took detailed notes. Diagnostic criteria were rated after the interview was completed and the interviewer had also examined available chart materials. Items are scored 'not present', 'subthreshold', 'present', and 'strongly present'. The interviewer must have clear evidence for the presence of a criterion as a stable characteristic of the patient — it must have been present during at least the preceding five years, not restricted to periods with Axis I disorders or to specific situations — to make a positive rating. For the present study, items were re-coded into two categories: 'absent' or 'present'. Categorical diagnoses and dimensional scores (i.e., total number of criteria present for each disorder) were derived. No interrater reliability data were collected for Axis II categorical diagnoses or dimensional ratings, but in most cases the scoring was reviewed by a second, senior-level clinical psychologist, who also knew the patient.

PROCEDURE

Since January 1996, newly admitted patients were assessed upon admission T1; baseline assessment) with a standardized psychological assessment battery. PCL-R psychopathy assessment was implemented in November 1997. In order to provide information on treatment progress, all patients in our hospital are re-tested 18-24 months after admission (T2), and again 42 months after admission (T3). At baseline, PCL-R and SIDP-R/SIDP-IV interviews were administered to assess PCL-R psychopathy and Axis II disorders. Because PCL-R psychopathy assessment was not implemented until November 1997, 26 patients were administered the PCL-R at T2. The examiner who diagnosed a particular patient using DSM-IV Axis II criteria was blind with respect to the PCL-R

---

[2] DSM-III-R Axis II diagnoses (SIDP-R interviews) were recoded into DSM-IV Axis II diagnoses.

psychopathy score of this particular patient. Occasionally, however, PCL-R examiners had
been in contact with the patient previously for other psychodiagnostic activities (especially
for patients who were administered the PCL-R at T2).

PCL-R and SIDP-R/SIDP-IV ratings were conducted by a pool of 10 examiners,
seven female and three male. Seven raters were master's level (clinical) psychologists, one
rater was an experienced Ph.D. clinical and forensic psychologist (CdR), one a mental
health scientist, and one rater had a degree in both mental health science and law (MH). All
were familiar with DSM-IV Axis I/Axis II disorders and were experienced in assessment
and/or treatment of (forensic) psychiatric patients.

## RESULTS

### PCL-R SCORES

Figure 1 presents the distribution of PCL-R psychopathy scores in the sample. The
mean total PCL-R score (adjusted sum) was 21.4 ($SD$ = 8.4), with a range from 3 to 38, a
median score of 21.1 and a mode of 17. The kurtosis of the PCL-R total score was $-.753$
(SE = -.244). PCL-R scores were normally distributed (Kolmogorov-Smirnov $Z$ = .594, $p$ =
.872). The mean Factor 1 score was 9.3 ($SD$ = 3.8) and the mean Factor 2 score was also
9.3 ($SD$ = 5.0). When we applied a cut-off point of 26, which is often used in European
research (Grann, Längström, Tengström, Stålenheim, 1998; Rasmussen et al., 1999), to
divide the patients into a psychopathic and a nonpsychopathic group, 34 patients (34.7%)
were classified as 'psychopaths'. When a threshold of 30, designated by Hare (1991), was
used, 21 (21.4%) of the patients received a diagnosis of psychopathy. Nine patients (9.2%)
had very low scores (PCL-R score < 10).

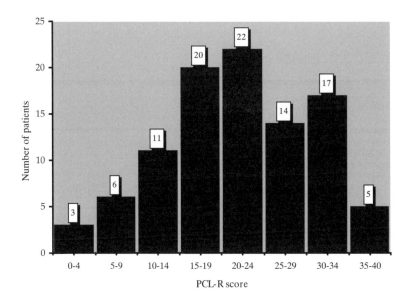

**Figure 1**
*Distribution of PCL-R Psychopathy Scores (N = 98)*

**AXIS I DISORDERS**

There was a high frequency of psychiatric disorders in the study sample. Table 1 presents base rates of lifetime Axis I disorders.

TABLE 1
*Base Rate of DSM-IV Axis I Disorders (N = 98)*

| Diagnosis | *n* | % |
|---|---|---|
| Organic brain syndrome | 2 | 2.0 |
| Schizophrenia/other psychotic disorder | 17 | 17.3 |
| Mood disorders | 5 | 5.1 |
|   Depressive disorder not otherwise specified | 3 | 3.1 |
|   Bipolar disorder | 2 | 2.0 |
| Anxiety disorders | 4 | 4.1 |
|   Anxiety disorder not otherwise specified | 2 | 2.0 |
|   Posttraumatic stress disorder | 1 | 1.0 |
|   Social phobia | 1 | 1.0 |
| Sedative, hypnotic, anxiolytic abuse/dependence disorders | 5 | 5.1 |
| Alcohol use disorders | 27 | 27.6 |
|   Alcohol abuse/dependence | 25 | 25.5 |
|   Alcohol intoxication | 1 | 1.0 |
|   Alcohol withdrawal | 1 | 1.0 |
| Psychoactive substance abuse/dependence disorders | 46 | 46.9 |
|   Cannabis | 16 | 16.3 |
|   Polysubstance | 10 | 10.2 |
|   Cocaine abuse | 8 | 8.2 |
|   Unknown/other substance | 6 | 6.1 |
|   Amphetamine | 2 | 2.0 |
|   Opiod | 3 | 3.1 |
|   Hallucinogen | 1 | 1.0 |
| Paraphilias | 20 | 20.4 |
|   Pedophilia | 15 | 15.3 |
|   Parafilia not otherwise specified | 4 | 4.1 |
|   Exhibitionism | 1 | 1.0 |
| Pathological gambling | 11 | 11.2 |
| Other | 14 | 14.3 |
| Other | 14 | 14.3 |
| Any Axis I disorder | 86 | 87.8 |
| Any Axis I disorder (other than alcohol, substance or sedative abuse/dependence) | 61 | 62.2 |

Eighty-six patients (88%) met criteria for at least one Axis I disorder, including any alcohol or other substance related disorder (i.e., psychoactive substance, or sedative use disorders). Sixty-one patients (62%) met criteria for an Axis I diagnosis other than alcohol or psychoactive substance related disorders. Forty-seven patients (48%) met criteria for at least one substance related disorder. In addition, 20 patients (20%) received a diagnosis of paraphilia; 17 patients (17%) met criteria for schizophrenia or another psychotic disorder; 11 patients (11%) received a diagnosis of pathological gambling, five met criteria for a mood disorder, four of an anxiety disorder, and two of an organic brain syndrome. Other diagnoses ($n$ = 14) included impulse control disorder ($n$ = 4), pervasive developmental disorder NOS ($n$ = 2), pyromania ($n$ = 2), attention-deficit/hyperactivity disorder ($n$ = 2), Asperger's disorder, autistic disorder, Gilles de la Tourette, and hypochondriasis (all $n$ = 1).

**AXIS II DISORDERS**

Valid data were obtained from 94 patients. The prevalence of personality disorders in the sample was substantial (Table 2). Eighty-four patients (89%) received at least one Axis II diagnosis. Of the remaining 10 patients, two received a SIDP-IV diagnosis "mixed PD", defined as missing only one criterion for two or more PDs. Thus, only eight patients did not receive a PD diagnosis. Co-morbidity on Axis II was more common than a single diagnosis: of the 83 patients given a PD diagnosis, 53 (64%) received multiple diagnoses. The mean number of PDs per patient, for patients with at least one PD was 2.1. As expected, most PDs are found in Cluster B disorders, followed by Cluster A. The most frequently diagnosed PD was antisocial PD ($n$ = 45), followed by narcissistic ($n$ = 26), borderline ($n$ = 24), and paranoid PD ($n$ = 18).

Co-morbidity between lifetime Axis I and Axis II disorder diagnoses was high. Seventy-one patients (72%) with at least one PD diagnosis did have at least one (lifetime) Axis I disorder diagnosis (including alcohol/drug/sedative use disorders). When alcohol/drug use disorders were excluded from the analyses, 49 patients (50%) met criteria for both Axis I and Axis II disorder diagnoses.

TABLE 2
*Base Rate of DSM-IV Axis II Diagnoses and Mean Dimensional Scores (N = 94)*

| Personality disorder | Categorical diagnoses | | Number of traits present | |
|---|---|---|---|---|
| | *n* | % | Mean | *SD* |
| Paranoid | 18 | 19.1 | 1.89 | 1.76 |
| Schizoid | 7 | 7.4 | 1.09 | 1.37 |
| Schizotypal | 9 | 9.6 | 1.70 | 1.96 |
| Antisocial | 45 | 47.8 | — | — |
| Conduct disorder (< 15 years) | 55 | 58.5 | 3.88 | 2.29 |
| Antisocial behavior since age 15 | 66 | 70.2 | 3.73 | 3.37 |
| Borderline | 24 | 25.5 | 2.79 | 2.44 |
| Histrionic | 5 | 5.3 | 0.95 | 1.35 |
| Narcissistic | 26 | 27.7 | 2.94 | 2.42 |
| Avoidant | 11 | 11.7 | 1.24 | 1.83 |
| Dependent | 4 | 4.3 | 1.09 | 1.60 |
| Obsessive-compulsive | 9 | 9.6 | 1.53 | 1.40 |
| Passive-aggressive | 7 | 7.4 | 1.15 | 1.45 |
| Self-defeating | 4 | 4.3 | 1.33 | 1.63 |
| Depressive | 6 | 7.2 | 1.31 | 1.32 |
| Cluster A | 29 | 30.9 | — | — |
| Cluster B | 66 | 70.2 | — | — |
| Cluster C | 22 | 23.4 | — | — |
| Any personality disorder (mixed excluded) | 84 | 89.3 | — | — |

*Note.* For depressive personality disorder, $N = 83$. '—' = not calculated.

## CATEGORICAL OVERLAP AXIS I / AXIS II DISORDERS WITH PCL-R PSYCHOPATHY

It is apparent from Table 1 and Table 2 that several diagnostic categories have (very) low base rates. Therefore, following Hart and Hare (1989), we excluded diagnostic categories with fewer than 10 patients from further analyses (i.e., base rate < 10%). This resulted in 10 categories, five Axis I (schizophrenia, alcohol abuse/dependence, other substance abuse/dependence, paraphilias, pathological gambling), and five Axis II (paranoid, antisocial, borderline, narcissistic, and avoidant PD). Cluster A, B, and C disorders (presence of at least one PD of the particular Cluster), and any Axis I, any Axis II

were also included as diagnostic categories. Patients were divided into a low (PCL-R <
20), a medium ($20 \leq$ PCL-R < 30) and a high (PCL-R $\geq$ 30) psychopathy group. The chi-
square test was used to determine differences in frequency distribution between diagnostic
categories. In addition, we calculated odds ratios from $2 \times 2$ (presence vs. absence of
diagnosis) tables. An odds ratio refers to the conditional probability of disorder A (i.e.,
PCL-R psychopathy) given that another disorder B (e.g., schizophrenia) is present, divided
by the conditional probability of disorder A given that disorder B is not present (Fleiss,
1981). Odds ratios of 2 or 3 are typically considered to indicate a large effect size (Fleiss,
Williams, & Dubro, 1986). Odds ratios were calculated for the recommended cut-off point
of 30 to form psychopathic and nonpsychopathic groups, as well as for the cut-off point of
26. The chi-square statistic was used to determine the significance of each odds ratio
(Fleiss, 1981). To reduce the risk of chance capitalization, Bonferroni correction (Stevens,
1986) is used for the chi-square tests. We tested each Axis separately. Because there were
five comparisons for Axis I disorders, the Type 1 error rate per individual test was set at
.01. For Axis II, there were eight comparisons, and the Type 1 error rate per individual test
was set at .006.

With regard to the overlap between PCL-R psychopathy and Axis I disorders, we
found a significant association between drug use disorders and PCL-R psychopathy [$\chi^2$ (2,
98) = 9.51, $p$ = .009]. For alcohol use related disorders, we found a positive trend [$\chi^2$ (2,
98) = 5.70, $p$ = .058]. Paraphilia and any Axis I diagnosis showed a trend towards a
negative associations with PCL-R psychopathy [$\chi^2$ (2, 98) = 6.22, $p$ = .045 and $\chi^2$(2, 98)
= 7.11, $p$ = .029, respectively].

The odds ratios indicate that a diagnosis of PCL-R psychopathy (total score $\geq$ 30)
was positively associated with drug abuse/dependence and alcohol abuse/dependence. On
the other hand, the odds ratio indicated that patients with a diagnosis of PCL-R
psychopathy were about three and a half times less likely to receive a diagnosis of any
Axis I disorder other than alcohol or other substance use disorders. Similarly, these
patients were about three times less likely to receive a diagnosis of paraphilias.

With regard to Axis II diagnoses, high PCL-R scores were significantly associated
with Cluster B disorders [$\chi^2$ (2, 94) = 18.55, $p$ < .001]. More specifically, high PCL-R

scores tended to be significantly associated with antisocial PD [$\chi^2$ (2, 94) = 17.77, $p$ < .001]. In fact, 88% of patients with a PCL-R score ≥ 26 had a DSM-IV antisocial PD; the reverse was not true. Also, there were trends for paranoid [$\chi^2$ (2, 94) = 7.78, $p$ = .020], borderline [$\chi^2$ (2, 94) = 5.01, $p$ = .082), and any PD [$\chi^2$ (2, 94) = 9.46, $p$ = .009].

Finally, computation of positive predictive power (PPP) (Widiger, Hurt, Frances, Clarkin, & Gilmore, 1984), defined as the conditional probability of having one disorder given the other, strongly indicated that a diagnosis of PCL-R psychopathy was highly predictive of antisocial PD (PPP = 0.85). The reverse was not true: a diagnosis of antisocial PD did not predict PCL-R psychopathy (PPP = 0.38). The association between PCL-R psychopathy and Axis I and Axis II categorical diagnoses is summarized in Table 3.

TABLE 3
*Patients with Low ( < 20), Medium (20-29) and High (≥ 30) PCL-R Scores Diagnosed with Axis I and Axis II Categorical Diagnoses, and Association (odds ratio) Between Categorical Diagnoses of PCL-R Psychopathy and DSM-IV Disorders*

| Diagnostic category[a] | PCL-R score | | | | Odds ratio[c] | |
|---|---|---|---|---|---|---|
| | < 20 | 20-29 | ≥ 30 | $p$[b] | PCL-R ≥ 26 | PCL-R ≥ 30 |
| **Axis I diagnosis** | | | | | | |
| Schizophrenia | 6 | 9 | 2 | .316 | .55 | .44 |
| No Schizophrenia | 34 | 28 | 19 | | | |
| Alcohol abuse/dependence | 6 | 10 | 9 | .058 | 2.29 | 2.86 |
| No alcohol | 34 | 27 | 12 | | | |
| Drug abuse/dependence | 9 | 16 | 13 | **.009** | **2.70** | 3.38 |
| No drug abuse/dependence | 31 | 21 | 8 | | | |
| Paraphilias | 13 | 5 | 2 | .045 | .28 | .35 |
| No paraphilias | 27 | 32 | 19 | | | |

*(table continues)*

TABLE 3 (cont.)

| Diagnostic category[a] | PCL-R score | | | $p$[b] | Odds ratio[c] | |
|---|---|---|---|---|---|---|
| | < 20 | 20-29 | ≥ 30 | | PCL-R ≥ 26 | PCL-R ≥ 30 |
| Pathological gambling | 5 | 3 | 3 | .732 | 1.76 | 1.44 |
| No pathological gambling | 35 | 34 | 18 | | | |
| Any Axis I[d] | 29 | 24 | 8 | .029 | .42 | .28 |
| No Axis I | 11 | 13 | 13 | | | |
| **Axis II diagnosis** | | | | | | |
| Paranoid PD | 3 | 7 | 8 | .020 | 2.88 | 3.88 |
| No paranoid PD | 34 | 29 | 13 | | | |
| Antisocial PD | 9 | 19 | 17 | **<.001** | **20.39** | **6.83** |
| No antisocial PD | 28 | 17 | 4 | | | |
| Borderline PD | 6 | 9 | 9 | .082 | 2.33 | 2.90 |
| No borderline PD | 31 | 27 | 12 | | | |
| Narcissistic PD | 6 | 13 | 7 | .132 | 2.40 | 1.53 |
| No narcissistic PD | 31 | 23 | 14 | | | |
| Avoidant PD | 6 | 4 | 1 | .423 | .66 | .32 |
| No avoidant PD | 31 | 32 | 20 | | | |
| Cluster A | 8 | 12 | 9 | .223 | 1.19 | 1.99 |
| No cluster A | 29 | 24 | 12 | | | |
| Cluster B | 17 | 29 | 20 | **<.001** | **25.41** | **11.74** |
| No cluster B | 20 | 7 | 1 | | | |
| Cluster C | 10 | 10 | 2 | .233 | .63 | .28 |
| No cluster C | 27 | 26 | 19 | | | |
| Any personality disorder (mixed PD not included) | 28 | 35 | 20 | **.009** | **6.28** | 3.18 |
| No personality disorder | 9 | 1 | 1 | | | |

*Note.* PD = personality disorder. For Axis I disorders, $N = 98$, for Axis II disorders, $N = 94$. Significant (Bonferroni corrected) values are in bold.
[a] Diagnostic categories ≥ 10 patients (see text). [b,c] Chi-square test. [d] Other than alcohol or psychoactive substance use disorder diagnoses.

### DIMENSIONAL OVERLAP AXIS II DISORDERS WITH PCL-R PSYCHOPATHY

Product-moment correlations were used to examine the association between PCL-R scores and Axis II dimensional scores (see Table 4). Because there were 14 comparisons for Axis II dimensional scores, the Type 1 error rate per individual test was set at .004. Except for antisocial behavior since age 15, dimensional ratings of personality disorders were not normally distributed; we therefore subjected them to logarithmic transformation before computing correlations with PCL-R scores.

**TABLE 4**
*Correlations Between PCL-R Psychopathy Scores and Axis II Dimensional Scores (N = 94)*

| | PCL-R | | |
| Personality disorder | Total | Factor 1 | Factor 2 |
| --- | --- | --- | --- |
| Paranoid | **.44**$^{**}$ | **.36**$^{**}$ | **.38**$^{**}$ |
| Schizoid | -.14 | -.02 | -.18 |
| Schizotypal | .04 | .07 | .01 |
| Conduct disorder (< 15 years) | **.53**$^{**}$ | **.30**$^{*}$ | **.58**$^{**}$ |
| Antisocial behavior since age 15 | **.64**$^{**}$ | **.39**$^{**}$ | **.65**$^{**}$ |
| Borderline | **.33**$^{*}$ | .20 | **.32**$^{*}$ |
| Histrionic | **.32**$^{*}$ | **.37**$^{**}$ | .15 |
| Narcissistic | **.47**$^{**}$ | **.57**$^{**}$ | .26 |
| Avoidant | -.19 | -.18 | -.16 |
| Dependent | -.02 | -.04 | .00 |
| Obsessive-compulsive | .19 | .27 | .04 |
| Passive-aggressive | .28 | .16 | **.32**$^{*}$ |
| Self-defeating | .19 | -.06 | **.31**$^{*}$ |
| Depressive | -.13 | -.18 | -.06 |

*Note.* For depressive personality disorder, $N = 83$. Significant values (Bonferroni corrected) values are in bold.
$^{*}p < .004.$ $^{**}p < .001.$

Correlations with dimensional ratings revealed a strong association of the PCL-R total score with six Axis II disorders: PCL-R total scores correlated positively and significantly ($r \geq .32$) with paranoid PD, conduct disorder (< 15 years), antisocial behavior since age 15, borderline, histrionic, and narcissistic PD. The difference between PCL-R Factor 1 and Factor 2 was quite pronounced. Factor 1 showed significant positive correlations ≥ .30 for paranoid, histrionic and narcissistic PD, and also for conduct disorder (< 15 years) and antisocial behavior after age 15. Factor 2 correlated positively ($r ≥ .31$) with self-defeating, passive-aggressive, borderline and paranoid PD, and also with conduct disorder and antisocial behavior since age 15. Thus, only paranoid PD, conduct disorder (< 15 years) and antisocial behavior since age 15 were significantly and meaningfully related to both factors of the PCL-R. Neither factor correlated with schizoid, schizotypal, avoidant, dependent, obsessive-compulsive, and depressive PD.

## DISCUSSION

In general, a high prevalence of lifetime DSM-IV Axis I psychiatric morbidity was found in the study sample. Almost 88% of the sample met criteria for at least one Axis I disorder, including any alcohol or substance related disorder. The finding that substance use disorders were the most prevalent type of disorder is consistent with most other studies with forensic subjects (Hart & Hare, 1989 Stålenheim & von Knorring, 1996; Timmerman & Emmelkamp, 2001). However, only five percent of our patients were diagnosed with a lifetime diagnosis of a mood disorder, which is rather low compared to other studies with forensic psychiatric patients (Côté & Hodgins, 1992; Hart & Hare, 1989; Stålenheim & von Knorring, 1996; Timmerman & Emmelkamp, 2001). Timmerman and Emmelkamp (2001), for example, found that 51% of a sample ($N = 37$) of Dutch TBS patients had a lifetime diagnosis of affective disorder. In their study, Axis I diagnoses were based on a fully structured interview, whereas in the present study Axis I diagnoses were mainly based on file information, which may have resulted in an underestimation of the real psychopathology.  On the other hand, prevalence rates for affective disorders typically range from about three to 25%, in different forensic settings (Eaves, Tien, & Wilson, 2000).

The high percentage of patients with a PD that we found, is comparable to prevalence rates between 60 and 80% in other European forensic psychiatric samples (Blackburn, Crellin, Morgan, & Tulloch, 1990; Coid, 1992; Kullgren, Grann, & Holmberg, 1996). De Ruiter and Greeven (2000), for example, found that 80% of a Dutch sample of 85 forensic psychiatric patients fulfilled diagnostic criteria for at least one PD according to the SIDP-R, with paranoid, antisocial, borderline and narcissistic PD the most prevalent. Timmerman and Emmelkamp (2001) reported a lower frequency of PDs (45%) in a rather small sample ($N$ = 39) of Dutch forensic psychiatric patients. The difference is probably due to the fact that in the present study, as in the study by de Ruiter and Greeven (2000), the interviewers also reviewed file records consisting of elaborate psychiatric and psychological evaluations, criminal history records, and family background data, whereas in the Timmerman and Emmelkamp (2001) study, PD diagnoses were based exclusively on information obtained from the patient, which most likely led to an underestimation of the prevalence of certain PDs. Indeed, de Ruiter and Greeven (2000) reported that especially Cluster B disorders are more difficult to detect by means of a self-report instrument, compared to a semi-structured interview, because of the lack of self-insight and defensiveness inherent to Cluster B disorders. In line with these findings, Zimmerman and Coryell (1990) found that histrionic and antisocial PD were more often diagnosed on the basis of a semi-structured interview than with a self-report questionnaire. In our view, the use of a semi-structured interview in combination with extensive collateral information is indispensable for the diagnosis of PDs in forensic subjects.

An alternative explanation for the lower frequency of PDs in the sample of Timmerman and Emmelkamp (2001) might be that, originally, TBS patients were referred to a *specific* hospital (e.g., the Dr. Henri van der Hoeven Kliniek) *after* having been examined in a special selection institute, where the best treatment program for their needs was decided. This selection might have caused differences between the patient populations between the forensic psychiatric institutions. At the present time, random selection is practiced.

The PCL-R mean scores and standard deviations in our sample are comparable to those that have been reported in other European samples (Cooke, 1998; Logan, Blackburn, Donelly, & Renwick, 2002), as is the proportion of patients classified as psychopaths (Stålenheim & von Knorring, 1996). Our findings suggest that high PCL-R scores tend to be positively associated with Axis I drug abuse/dependence, and negatively (trends) with schizophrenia and its variants, paraphilias and any Axis I disorder (other than alcohol/drug use disorders). The results are consistent with findings of earlier studies (Hart & Hare, 1986; Nedopil et al., 1998; Rasmussen et al., 1996; Stålenheim & von Knorring, 1996).

In addition, the PCL-R showed a clear and expected pattern of associations with Axis II disorders. A PCL-R diagnosis was most strongly and significantly associated with a diagnosis of antisocial PD. This finding is consistent with existing findings on the construct validity of the PCL(-R) in a variety of populations, including North American male prisoners (Harpur, Hare, & Hakstian, 1989) and forensic psychiatric patients (Hart & Hare, 1989), as well as European samples of forensic psychiatric patients (Blackburn, 1998a; Stålenheim & von Knorring, 1996). Also consistent with previous research (Hart & Hare, 1989; Stålenheim & von Knorring, 1996), we found that the link between PCL-R psychopathy and antisocial PD is asymmetric. Most patients (81%) diagnosed as psychopaths by PCL-R criteria met criteria for a diagnosis of antisocial PD, whereas a minority (38%) of those with antisocial PD also received a diagnosis of PCL-R psychopathy.

Correlations between PCL-R scores and dimensional scores of Axis II disorders demonstrated positive correlations $\geq$ .32 of the PCL-R total score with six of the 13 disorders. These findings are largely consistent with previous findings (Blackburn, 1998a; Hare, 1991; Hart & Hare, 1989; Hart, Hare, & Forth, 1994; Stålenheim & von Knorring, 1996), as is the significant correlation of Factor 1 with paranoid and antisocial, histrionic and narcissistic dimensional scores, and the positive correlation of Factor 2 with paranoid and antisocial dimensional scores (Blackburn, 1998a). However, Hart and Hare (1989) found that Factor 2 correlated significantly only with antisocial PD, which may be due to the lower base rate of psychopathy (12.5%) in the Hart and Hare sample. Of course, findings are in line with expectations, given the fact that a number of diagnostic criteria for these PDs are similar to a number of PCL-R criteria (e.g., grandiose sense of self-worth; impulsivity).

Several methodological limitations deserve attention. A limitation of our study is the fact that some of the Axis I diagnoses may not have been as reliable and valid as we would have liked them to be. The use of a (semi-)structured interview for the assessment of lifetime Axis I diagnoses according to the DSM-IV in combination with a record review would have been preferable. However, limited staff necessitated us to choose either an Axis I or Axis II semi-structured interview. Because patient files tended to include quite detailed information on Axis I pathology, we opted to employ the Axis II interview.

Second, Axis I and Axis II diagnoses, and PCL-R ratings were not completely independent from one another for all patients. Occasionally, raters had been in contact with the patient previously for other assessment sessions. This is especially true for some patients who were administered the PCL-R at T1. However, none of the raters had a long-term psychotherapeutic contact with a patient. We attempted to minimize bias in all cases, by using as a final PCL-R diagnosis a consensus between (at least) two independent PCL-R ratings.

To summarize, PCL-R psychopathy was significantly (Bonferroni corrected) positively related to non-alcohol substance use disorders, antisocial, and Cluster B PD. PCL-R scores were also positively correlated ($r \geq .30$) with dimensional scores of paranoid, borderline, and narcissistic PD, and with conduct disorder and antisocial behavior since age 15. In general, results are consistent with previous research, providing further evidence for the cross-cultural stability of the PCL-R.

Chapter 5

PSYCHOPATHY

PREDICTS INSTITUTIONAL MISBEHAVIOR[1]

[1] A slightly different version of this chapter is published as:
Hildebrand, M., Ruiter, C. de, & Nijman, H. (2004). PCL-R psychopathy predicts disruptive behavior among male offenders in a Dutch forensic psychiatric hospital. *Journal of Interpersonal Violence*, *19*, 13-29.
Thanks are due to Marleen Nagtegaal, Lieveken Vester and Vivienne de Vogel for assisting in data collection. We are grateful to Cécile Vandeputte-van de Vijver who assisted in establishing DSM-IV Axis I diagnoses.

## SUMMARY

The purpose of this research was to study the predictive validity of the Dutch language version of Hare's Psychopathy Checklist-Revised (PCL-R) by examining the relationship between PCL-R scores and various types of disruptive behavior during inpatient forensic psychiatric treatment. A sample of 92 male forensic psychiatric patients were rated on the PCL-R. From daily hospital information bulletins, incidents of verbal abuse, verbal threat, physical violence and violation of hospital rules were derived. Also, the number of seclusion episodes was recorded. As expected, significant correlations were found between PCL-R scores and verbal abuse, verbal threat, violation of rules, total number of incidents, and frequency of seclusion. Psychopaths (PCL-R $\geq$ 26) were significantly more often involved in incidents than nonpsychopaths. Multiple regression analyses revealed that the PCL-R Factor 2 score in particular contributed uniquely to the prediction of the total number of incidents. The findings are discussed in terms of their clinical implications.

## INTRODUCTION

Inpatient aggression threatens the safety and well being of staff members and patients, in both general psychiatric institutions (Ekblom, 1970; Lion & Reid, 1983; Nijman, Allertz, Merckelbach, à Campo, & Ravelli, 1997) and forensic hospitals (Litwack & Schlesinger, 1987). Studies indicate that about 15 - 30% of psychiatric patients engage in assaultive behavior during hospitalization (e.g., Karson & Bigelow, 1987; Nijman et al., 1997). Nursing staff in particular are at risk of being victimized (e.g., Nijman et al., 1997; Shah, Fineberg, & James, 1991). Apart from its physical and psychological consequences, inpatient aggression has considerable financial implications. Hunter and Carmel (1992), for example, reported an annual total of 134 serious injuries in a 973-bed forensic psychiatric hospital. The average cost per injury was conservatively estimated to be $ 5,719, resulting in a total annual loss of $766,290. Given its far-reaching consequences, aggression prevention in (forensic) psychiatric inpatient facilities should have high priority. For effective prevention, however, it is important that clinicians can predict violent behavior in forensic psychiatric patients with sufficient accuracy (Harris & Rice, 1997). Insight into the factors associated with aggressive behavior in forensic psychiatric patients, is likely to increase the possibilities for staff to manage and prevent this behavior effectively.

Studies have revealed numerous risk factors associated with inpatient violence in (forensic) psychiatric patients (e.g. Ball, Young, Dotson, Brothers, & Robbins, 1994; Hare & McPerson, 1984; Monahan, 1981; Tardiff, 1997), including individual (e.g., age, ethnic origin, number of total prior convictions, psychotic disorder, drug/alcohol abuse, personality disorder) and situational (e.g., overcrowding, staff inexperience, management tolerance of violence) factors. However, the most important generalization that can be made from existing research on the relationship between patient characteristics and disruptive behavior within (forensic) psychiatric hospitals is that no strong relationships are known, except for a history of prior violence, which is regarded as the best predictor of aggression (e.g., Harris & Rice, 1997; Shah et al., 1991).

In the past two decades, the relationship between psychopathy, as defined by the Psychopathy Checklist-Revised (PCL-R; Hare, 1991) or its derivatives, and various forms of inpatient disruptive behavior (e.g., verbal aggression, physical violence, escape attempts) has been studied in a variety of (mainly North-American) samples of adult male prisoners and forensic psychiatric patients (Belfrage, Fransson, & Strand , 2000; Buffington-Vollum, Edens, Johnson, & Johnson, 2002; Cooke, 1995, 1997; Edens, Buffington-Vollum, Colwell, Johnson, & Johnson, 2002; Gacono, Meloy, Sheppard, Speth, & Roske, 1995; Hare & McPherson, 1984; Hare, Clark, Grann, & Thornton, 2000; Heilbrun et al., 1998; Kosson, Steuerwald, Forth, & Kirkhart, 1997; Kroner & Mills, 2001; Moltó, Poy, & Torrubia, 2000; Pham, Remy, Dailliet, & Lienard, 1998; Reiss, Grubin, & Meux, 1999; Rice, Harris, & Cormier 1992; Serin, 1991), female inmates (Salekin, Rogers, & Sewell, 1997), general psychiatric patients (Rasmussen & Levander, 1996), and adolescent offenders (Brandt, Kennedy, Patrick, & Curtin, 1997; Edens, Poythress, & Lilienfeld, 1999; Forth, Hart, & Hare, 1990; Gretton, McBride, Hare, O'Shaughnessy, & Kumka, 2001; Hicks, Rogers, & Cashel, 2000; Myers, Burket, & Harris, 1995; Rogers, Johansen, Chang, & Salekin, 1997).

Overall, these studies indicate that high PCL-R scores are significantly (albeit sometimes modestly) associated with (more) disruptive behavior during hospitalization or imprisonment. With regard to acts of *physical* violence, however, remarkably divergent results have been found. Most recent studies report non-significant or below .20 correlations between psychopathy and physical violence in adult samples (e.g., Edens et al., 1999; Heilbrun et al., 1998; see Edens, Petrila, & Buffington-Vollum, in press, for a review of the literature).

While the literature that addresses the association between psychopathy and inpatient disruptive behavior is rapidly expanding, to the best of our knowledge, only a handful of studies have examined the relationship in forensic psychiatric patients. For example, Rice, Harris, and Cormier (1992; see also Harris, Rice, & Cormier, 1991) evaluated a therapeutic community treatment program in a forensic hospital in Ontario, Canada. Patients and controls were assessed with the PCL-R on the basis of file information only, and subsequently divided into a high (PCL-R > 25) and a low (PCL-R $\leq$ 25) psychopathy group. Comparisons between the groups indicated that patients with high scores displayed more behavior problems during treatment, including more episodes of seclusion during the first and last year of treatment.

Gacono et al. (1995) examined the association between PCL-R scores and behavior problems in hospitalized insanity acquittees. All insanity acquittees who malingered their psychiatric disorders successfully ($n$ = 18), scored 30 or more on the PCL-R. They also created significantly more institutional management problems (verbal or physical aggression, higher escape risk, and drugs dealing drugs), as compared to 18 insanity non-malingering comparison subjects.

Hill et al. (1996) studied the validity of the screening version of the PCL-R (PCL:SV; Hart, Cox, & Hare, 1995) as a predictor of institutional management problems in a sample of 55 adult offenders admitted to a maximum security forensic psychiatric institution in Texas. A six-month follow-up review of subjects' files was conducted, in which data on self-harm (frequency of suicide attempts and self-mutilation), aggression (verbal abuse, verbal threats, irritability, belligerence, fighting), escape potential (escape attempts and threats to escape) and treatment noncompliance (e.g., refusal of medication) were collected. Results indicated that the PCL:SV was predictive of aggression and treatment noncompliance. It was found that more than 35% of the physical aggression exhibited by nonpsychopaths was self-directed, while none of the psychopaths engaged in self-harming behavior.

Finally, Heilbrun et al. (1998) examined the relationship between PCL psychopathy and aggression in 218 mentally disordered offenders admitted to the Forensic Service, Florida State Hospital. Patients' hospital charts were reviewed for the first and last two months of hospitalization. Although significant correlations were found between total number of aggressive incidents and PCL total ($r$ = .30), Factor 1 ($r$ = .24), and Factor 2 ($r$ = .25) scores during the first two months of hospitalization, this association was no longer significant during the last two months of hospitalization (no $r$'s reported), which may be an indication that the institutional behavior of patients with high PCL-R scores can change by altering environmental and situational factors (in a similar vein, see Cooke, 1997; Hare et al., 2000).

## THE PRESENT STUDY

Although past findings have been promising, further research is needed to study the predictive validity of the PCL-R with regard to inpatient disruptive behavior, especially among forensic psychiatric patients. In the present prospective study, the strength of the association was examined in a sample of Dutch forensic psychiatric inpatients. It is one of the first studies with a European (non-English) edition of the PCL-R. On the basis of the previous research discussed above, we hypothesized that:

(1)   High PCL-R scores are associated with higher frequencies of verbal aggression (i.e., verbal abuse, verbal threats);

(2)   High psychopathy subjects are more likely to violate hospital rules than low psychopathy subjects;

(3)   As a result of their disruptive behavior, subjects with high PCL-R scores will be more likely to be secluded. Seclusion is a procedure to prevent patients from harming themselves or their environment, when all other measures have failed. Seclusion may also be used at the patient's request in order to prevent overstimulation.

We also considered a number of demographic and clinical variables as potentially related to inpatient aggression in order to compare the PCL-R with other predictors of inpatient aggression. These variables included age, ethnic origin, number of prior convictions, the presence or absence of a lifetime DSM-IV Axis I diagnosis of psychotic disorder, alcohol abuse/dependence, substance use disorder, and presence/absence of Axis II diagnoses of antisocial and borderline personality disorder (PD). The selection of the variables was based on both empirical (suggested by previous research, e.g., Ball et al., 1994; Tardiff, 1997) and practical (availability) considerations.

# METHOD

## SETTING

The study was conducted at the Dr. Henri van der Hoeven Kliniek, a forensic psychiatric hospital for residential treatment of mentally disordered criminal offenders in the Netherlands. According to Dutch criminal law, a criminal offender can be sentenced to a *maatregel van terbeschikkingstelling* (TBS-order) when (1) the offense committed can result in a sentence of four or more years of imprisonment, with an estimated high risk of recurrence, and (2) as a consequence of his mental condition the offender is judged to carry diminished responsibility for the offense. The main purpose of the TBS-order is to protect society from unacceptable high risks of recidivism, directly through involuntary admission to a forensic psychiatric hospital, and indirectly by offering treatment to the mentally disordered offender. Treatment is aimed at structural and lasting behavior change, thus allowing a safe return to society. Every one or two years the court reviews the risk of re-offending to determine whether the TBS-order needs to be prolonged (for more details, see Chapter 2).

## SAMPLE CHARACTERISTICS

The sample consisted of 92 male forensic psychiatric patients admitted to the Dr. Henri van der Hoeven Kliniek between January 1996 and July 2001. The mean age at admission for the sample was 31 years ($SD$ = 7.4; range = 19 - 50). Half of the sample was convicted for (attempted) murder or manslaughter, 26% for sexual offenses (e.g., assault, child molest, rape), and 17% for (aggravated) assault. In terms of ethnic origin, 77% of the patients were White.

The Dutch language version (van den Brink & de Jong, 1992) of the Structured Interview for Disorders of Personality (SIDP-R; Pfohl, Blum, Zimmerman, & Stangl, 1989) or its modified version (SIDP-IV; Pfohl, Blum, & Zimmerman, 1995; Dutch translation: de Jong, Derks, van Oel, & Rinne, 1996) was used for the assessment of PDs. Our initial use of DSM-III-R Axis II criteria is a consequence of the duration of the data collection phase, which started before the Dutch version of the SIDP-IV was available. Eleven patients were diagnosed using DSM-III-R criteria; the rest was diagnosed using

DSM-IV criteria. Seventy-five patients (i.e., 83%; two missing SIDP-R assessments) met the criteria for one or more PDs. In particular, Cluster B ('dramatic-erratic-emotional') PDs were frequently diagnosed: 45 patients (50%) received a diagnosis of antisocial PD, 25 narcissistic PD (28%), and 23 patients (26%) were diagnosed with a borderline PD. Paranoid PD (Cluster A) was also highly prevalent in this sample (i.e., 17 patients or 19%).

Lifetime DSM-IV Axis I diagnoses for psychotic disorder and alcohol/psychoactive substance use disorder diagnoses (present vs. absent) were coded by the primary author (MH) on the basis of all available data (e.g., earlier psychological and psychiatric reports, current psychiatric and psychological assessments). A senior-diagnostician and a senior clinical psychologist (CdR) reviewed all diagnoses and final diagnoses were reached in a consensus meeting. Fourteen patients (16%) met criteria for a (lifetime) DSM-IV Axis I psychotic disorder. Twenty-three patients (25%) met criteria for at least one (lifetime) Axis I alcohol use disorder (abuse/dependence) and 35 patients (38%) received a diagnosis of Axis I psychoactive substance abuse/dependence.

## PROCEDURE

*Assessment of psychopathy.* Within the first six weeks of admission, patients were administered a standard battery of psychological tests which included the PCL-R to assess psychopathy. The PCL-R is a reliable, well-validated (e.g., Hare et al., 2000; Hart, Hare, & Harpur, 1992; Hempill, Hare, & Wong, 1998) 20-item checklist based on traditional concepts of psychopathy (Cleckley, 1941/1982). The total score can range from 0 to 40, and represents the degree to which a subject resembles the prototypical psychopath (Hare, 1991). Factor analyses fairly consistently revealed a stable, oblique two-factor structure (e.g., Cooke & Michie, 1997; Hare, 1991; Hobson & Shine, 1998). Factor 1 has been described as 'callous and remorseless disregard for the rights and feelings of others'; Factor 2 has been labeled 'chronically unstable and antisocial lifestyle' (Hare, 1991).

PCL-R assessments were made on the basis of the Dutch language version of the semi-structured PCL-R interview and extensive file review, in accordance with recommendations in the PCL-R manual (Hare, 1991). Collateral information consisted of extensive psychiatric and psychological evaluations, police records, criminal history, and family background data. PCL-R items were scored on a three-point scale (0 = *item does not apply*, 1 = *uncertain, item applies to a certain extent*, 2 = *item definitively applies*) on the basis of the authorized Dutch language version of the Hare PCL-R manual (Vertommen, Verheul, de Ruiter, & Hildebrand, 2002). In a previous study (Hildebrand, de Ruiter, de Vogel, & van der Wolf, 2002), high interrater reliability was demonstrated for the Dutch language version of the PCL-R. The intraclass correlation coefficient of the PCL-R total score was .88 for a single rater (Factor 1 = .76; Factor 2 = .83). Ratings were also internally consistent (Cronbach's alpha for the PCL-R total score = .87). Factor scores used in subsequent analyses were computed by summing the ratings for the items composing Hare's (1991) two-factor solution.

Ten interviewers/raters conducted the PCL-R ratings: seven females and three males. Seven raters were (clinical) psychologists, one an experienced Ph.D. clinical and forensic psychologist (CdR), one a mental health scientist, and one rater had a degree in both mental health science and law (MH). All raters had been extensively trained in the PCL-R (see Chapter 3).

For 86 patients we had the disposal of *at least* two independent PCL-R ratings. We decided to obtain a final consensus rating for these 86 patients. These consensus scores are used in all subsequent statistical analyses. For the remaining six patients, PCL-R scores were based on the rating of a single rater (MH or CdR). The mean PCL-R total score (adjusted sum) for the 92 male patients in the present sample was 21.5 (*SD* = 8.5), with a range from 3 to 38. The mean Factor 1 score was 9.4 (*SD* = 3.9), for Factor 2 it was 9.7 (*SD* = 4.8). Thirty-three patients (36%) had PCL-R scores ≥ 26.

*Incidents*. Every day, the hospital's general coordinator on duty prepares a so-called 'information bulletin' to inform staff members and patients about unusual events (e.g., visitors from outside the hospital) and disruptive incidents (e.g., aggressive behavior, violations of hospital rules) during the last 24 hours in the hospital. Two raters (MH and HN) independently reviewed 35 randomly selected information bulletins to examine the degree of interrater agreement on whether the events reported (*n* = 153) were indeed incidents. It appeared that there was excellent agreement between the raters as to whether or not the reported events were incidents (Cohen's κ = .86; observed agreement = 93.5%).

Subsequently, we designed a classification scheme for assigning any incident to one of four categories: (1) *Verbal abuse* (e.g., cursing); (2) *Verbal threat* (e.g., threatening to stab someone with a knife); (3) *Physical violence* (e.g., hitting someone; smashing objects; self-harm); (4) *Violation of hospital rules* (e.g., use of drugs, possession of pornographic material; unauthorized absence). Three independent raters, including the first author, classified 100 randomly selected incidents described in the daily bulletins to examine interrater agreement, before all other information bulletins were coded. There was excellent agreement among the three raters with regard to type of incident (mean Cohen's $\kappa = .92$; observed agreement $= 92\%$). Following the interrater reliability check, daily information bulletins from January 22, 1996 (admission date of the first patient from this sample) until November 1, 2001 (end date study period) were coded by an independent research assistant. Incidents were rated as discrete events, and the total number of incidents in each category was obtained for each patient.

*Seclusion.* Computerized hospital case files were reviewed by MH for frequencies of seclusion (either in the patient's own room or in a room especially designated for isolating patients in order to control aggression and/or psychosis). Again, episodes of seclusion during the study period were coded as discrete events, and the total number of instances was recorded for each patient. Since length of hospital stay was not equal for patients (range from 3 to 64 months; mode $= 7$ months), all outcome variables were corrected for length of stay.

## STATISTICAL ANALYSES

Spearman $\rho$ correlations were calculated between PCL-R scores and all outcome variables. Student's *t*-test was used to test mean group differences between PCL-R psychopaths (adjusted PCL-R total score $\geq 26$) and nonpsychopaths (total score $< 26$) on the criterion variables. Given the *a priori* hypotheses being tested regarding the relationship between PCL-R scores and inpatient aggression and seclusion, one-tailed tests were employed in this study, except for the association between PCL-R score and PV (two-tailed test).

Finally, multiple regression analyses were conducted in order to determine how the PCL-R compared with other established (demographic and clinical) predictor variables. In addition to standard multiple regression analyses, hierarchical regression analyses were performed to determine if adding PCL-R psychopathy improved prediction of incidents above and beyond that of selected demographic and clinical variables.

## RESULTS

### FREQUENCY OF DISRUPTIVE BEHAVIOR

On average, the 92 patients stayed in the hospital for 34 months, excluding days of (un)authorized absence. During the study period (i.e., January 22, 1996 - November 1, 2001), a total of 825 incidents were identified. The average number of incidents per patient was 9.0 ($SD$ = 11.6, range 0 - 85). Only nine patients (10%) never displayed any type of incident as reported on the information bulletin. The mean frequency of incidents per patient per year was 3.2.

With regard to type of disruptive behavior, 259 of the 825 incidents (31%) concerned verbal abuse, 125 (15%) were verbal threats, and 74 (9%) involved physical violence. The remaining 367 incidents (44%) were violations of hospital rules, including episodes of unauthorized absence [14 patients (15%) had escaped from the hospital on one or more occasions during the study period]. Seventy-three patients (79%) had been secluded — either in their own room or in a special seclusion chamber — on a total of 587 occasions. As expected, the frequency of seclusion episodes was strongly related to the total number of incidents (Spearman $\rho$ = .62, $p$ < .01). The association with seclusion was significant for all types of disruptive behavior (Spearman $\rho$ correlations between .38 and .53, all $ps$ < .01).

### PCL-R SCORES IN RELATION TO DISRUPTIVE BEHAVIOR

Table 1 presents Spearman $\rho$ correlations between PCL-R scores and disruptive behavior and frequency of seclusion episodes.

TABLE 1
*Spearman ρ Correlations Between PCL-R Scores and Incidents and Seclusion*

| Type of Behavior | PCL-R total | Factor 1 | Factor 2 |
|---|---|---|---|
| Total number of incidents | .44** | .22** | .47** |
| Verbal abuse | .33** | .16 | .36** |
| Verbal threat | .45** | .35** | .37** |
| Physical violence | .03 | -.04 | .08 |
| Violations of hospital rules | .39** | .13 | .45** |
| Seclusion | .42** | .21* | .35** |

*Note.* PCL-R = Psychopathy Checklist-Revised.  Significant correlations are in bold.
$^*p < .05.$ $^{**}p < .01$ (all one-tailed, except for correlations between PCL-R scores and physical violence).

With regard to the total number of incidents, significant correlations were found for the PCL-R total ($r = .44, p < .01$), Factor 1 ($r = .22, p < .01$) and Factor 2 ($r = .47, p < .01$) scores. As to type of incident, verbal abuse was significantly related to the PCL-R total ($r = .33, p < .01$) and Factor 2 ($r = .36, p < .01$) score, whereas verbal threat related significantly to PCL-R total ($r = .45, p < .01$), Factor 1 ($r = .35, p < .01$) and Factor 2 ($r = .37, p < .01$) scores. Violation of hospital rules correlated significantly with the PCL-R total ($r = .39, p < .01$) and Factor 2 ($r = .45, p < .01$) score. No significant correlations were found between physical violence and PCL-R scores. The association between frequency of seclusion and PCL-R total ($r = .42, p = .05$), Factor 1 ($r = .21, p < .05$) and Factor 2 ($r = .35, p < .01$) scores was also significant. In general, Factor 2 correlations with disruptive behavior were higher than Factor 1 correlations.

Next, exploratory Kendall's tau correlational analyses were conducted in order to examine which *individual* PCL-R items were related to the total number of incidents. Fifteen of the 20 items were significantly correlated with the total number of incidents. The highest correlations were found for Item 3 (*Need for stimulation / proneness to boredom*; $r = .37, p < .01$), Item 14 (*Impulsivity*; $r = .36, p < .01$), Item 4 (*Pathological lying*; $r = .34, p < .01$) and Item 10 (*Poor behavioral controls*, $r = .32, p < .01$). Item 2 (*Grandiose sense of self-worth*), Item 7 (*Shallow affect*), Item 8 (*Callous / lack of empathy*), Item 11

(*Promiscuous sexual behavior*), and Item 16 (*Failure to accept responsibility for own actions*) were not significantly related to the total number of incidents.

PCL-R psychopaths versus nonpsychopaths. PCL-R psychopaths ($n$ = 33) were involved in 443 incidents (54%), with an average of 6.1 incidents per year, compared to 2.3 incidents per year for nonpsychopaths (Table 2). The difference is statistically significant [$t$ (90) = 3.21, $p$ < .01, one-tailed]. PCL-R psychopaths were significantly more often verbally abusive [$t$ (90) = 2.32, $p$ < .05, one-tailed] and threatening to others [$t$ (90) = 2.49, $p$ < .01, one-tailed] than nonpsychopaths. They also violated hospital rules more often [$t$ (90) = 3.44, $p$ < .01, one-tailed]. No significant differences were found with regard to physical violence. In addition, PCL-R psychopaths were also more frequently secluded [$t$ (90) = 3.16, $p$ < .01, one-tailed] than nonpsychopaths.

TABLE 2
*Mean Number of Incidents Per Year (standard deviation in parenthesis)*

| Type of Behavior | PCL-R score | | $p$ |
| --- | --- | --- | --- |
| | PCL-R ≥ 26 ($n$ = 33) | PCL-R < 26 ($n$ = 59) | |
| Total number of incidents | 6.1 (6.4) | 2.3 (2.8) | < .01 |
| Verbal abuse | 2.1 (3.3) | 0.7 (1.1) | < .05 |
| Verbal threat | 1.1 (1.8) | 0.3 (0.4) | < .01 |
| Physical violence | 0.5 (1.1) | 0.3 (0.9) | ns |
| Violations of hospital rules | 2.4 (1.9) | 1.1 1.3) | < .01 |
| Seclusion | 5.4 (6.0) | 1.8 (2.3) | < .01 |

*Note.* PCL-R = Psychopathy Checklist-Revised.

## REGRESSION ANALYSES

To uncover the relative contribution of different demographic and clinical variables to the frequency of total incidents, two stepwise multiple regression analyses were conducted. Predictor variables in the first analysis included age, ethnic origin (White versus other), number of prior convictions, and presence/absence of psychotic disorder, alcohol abuse/dependence, drug abuse/dependence, antisocial and borderline PD, as well as the PCL-R total score. In the second analysis, the PCL-R total score was replaced with the PCL-R factor scores.

In predicting the total number of incidents, the PCL-R total score accounted for 13% of the variance. At step 2, drug abuse/dependence added an $\Delta R^2$ of .06 (i.e., it accounted for 6% of the variance) to the prediction of the total number of incidents. In the second analysis (PCL-R total score replaced with PCL-R factor scores), the Factor 2 score was the only variable to enter the regression equation, accounting for 19% of the variance, making a significant contribution to the prediction of total number of incidents.

Next, as is summarized in Table 3, we conducted a series of stepwise regression analyses on the different incident categories that were significantly correlated with PCL-R Factor scores (i.e., verbal abuse, verbal threat and violation of rules, as well as seclusion episodes). The predictor variables included the demographic and clinical variables mentioned above, as well as the PCL-R Factor scores. Of these, alcohol abuse/dependence, drug abuse/dependence, antisocial and borderline PD, and PCL-R Factor 1 failed to enter any of the regression equations.

**TABLE 3**
*Multiple Regression Analyses for Institutional Misbehavior and Seclusion*

| Incident predictors | β | $\Delta R^2$ | $R^2$ |
|---|---|---|---|
| **Total number of incidents** | | | |
| Step 1: PCL-R Factor 2 | .44 | .19 | .19 |
| **Verbal abuse** | | | |
| Step 1: PCL-R Factor 2 | .16 | .12 | .12 |
| **Verbal threat** | | | |
| Step 1: PCL-R Factor 2 | .09 | .11 | .11 |
| Step 2: Ethnic origin (*0 = white, 1 = other*) | .69 | .05 | .16 |
| **Violation of hospital rules** | | | |
| Step 1: PCL-R Factor 2 | .15 | .17 | .17 |
| Step 2: Age | -.06 | .07 | .24 |
| **Seclusion** | | | |
| Step 1: Prior convictions | .22 | .14 | .14 |
| Step 2: Psychotic disorder (*0 = no, 1 = yes*) | 4.30 | .08 | .22 |
| Step 3: PCL-R Factor 2 | .26 | .05 | .27 |

*Note.* PCL-R = Psychopathy Checklist-Revised. $\Delta R^2$ = the amount of variance explained at each step. $R^2$ = the amount of variance explained cumulatively.

In predicting verbal abuse, the PCL-R Factor 2 score was the only significant predictor variable, accounting for (only) 12% of the variance. Factor 2 also contributed little to the prediction of verbal threat ($\Delta R^2$ = .11); ethnic origin added an $\Delta R^2$ of .05 to the prediction of verbal threat. In predicting violation of hospital rules, Factor 2 ($\Delta R^2$ = .17) and age ($\Delta R^2$ of .07; the younger, the more incidents) were significant predictors. With regard to frequency of seclusion, when Factor 2 was added at Step 3 (Step 1: prior convictions, $\Delta R^2$ = .14; Step 2: psychotic disorder, $\Delta R^2$ = .08), it substantially improved the prediction of seclusion ($\Delta R^2$ = .05).

Interestingly, even when all demographic and clinical variables were entered first (forced entry) at Step 1, and PCL-R scores were allowed to enter the model at Step 2 if they still could improve the prediction model significantly, both the PCL-R total and (in a separate analysis) the PCL-R Factor 2 score still contributed significantly to the prediction of total incidents.

## DISCUSSION

In forensic psychiatric patients, the level of PCL-R psychopathy has been demonstrated to be associated with the presence of a wide range of institutional misbehaviors and violence (e.g., Gacono et al., 1995; Heilbrun et al., 1998; Pham et al., 1998; Young, Justice, & Erdberg, 1999). In the present study, a clear relationship between PCL-R scores and disruptive behavior was observed; high psychopathy patients were involved in significantly more incidents. More specifically, verbal aggression (verbal abuse plus verbal threat) and violation of hospital rules were more characteristic of patients with high PCL-R scores than of patients with low PCL-R scores. In general, these findings are in line with earlier findings in forensic psychiatric patients (e.g., Hare & McPherson, 1984; Heilbrun et al., 1998; Hill et al., 1996) supporting the value of the PCL-R as a significant correlate of disruptive behavior in forensic inpatients.

The hypothesis that high PCL-R scorers would be more likely to be secluded than patients with low PCL-R scores was also supported. PCL-R psychopathy was significantly related to the frequency of seclusions as reported in computerized hospital files. This comes as no great surprise because seclusion is often preceded by an incident. It can be concluded that individuals scoring high on the PCL-R pose more managerial problems for hospital staff.

The PCL-R Factor 2 score appeared to be the most effective clinical variable for predicting the total number of incidents, as well as incidents of verbal abuse, verbal threat and violation of hospital rules, even when other factors related to disruptive behavior (e.g., age, number of prior convictions, psychotic disorder, antisocial PD) were taken into account. This suggests that the chronically unstable and socially deviant lifestyle factor is important to consider in forecasting and effectively managing different types of disruptive behavior. It should be noted, however, that the amount of variance accounted for appears to be relatively small (e.g., 19% for the total number of incidents) and may be of limited value for making assignments for individual patients. However, concentrating patients with high PCL-R scores on a specialized ward and a better understanding of their way of dealing with problems may reduce the frequency or severity of in-hospital incidents.

In the present study, PCL-R scores were not significantly related to incidents of physical violence. It should be noted, however, that the base rate of incidents for physical violence was rather low (9%), as was the total number of 825 registered incidents. The low base rate problem may to some extent account for the absence of predictive accuracy. Other researchers have also reported weak or non-significant relationships between PCL-R scores and physical violence incidents (e.g., Cooke, 1997; Heilbrun et al., 1998; Rasmussen & Levander, 1996), suggesting that environmental or situational factors that may inhibit the aggressive tendencies of persons who might be violent in less restrictive settings are important to consider (Buffington-Vollum et al., 2002). Furthermore, base-rates of (physical) inpatient aggression may change over time (e.g., Heilbrun et al., 1998; Ross, Hart, & Webster, 1998). Heilbrun et al. (1998) reported that, even though PCL scores were modestly predictive of physical aggression during the first two months of hospitalization, this pattern was not observed during the last two months rated. Hare et al. (2000), in a similar vein, reported data from a German hospital suggesting that changes in hospital policy and the introduction of special management strategies for patients with high PCL:SV scores reduced hospital violence. Our findings are also relevant from an economic point of view, since inpatient disruptive behavior may be related to a longer length of stay in the hospital and an increase in staff sick leaves (Nijman, 1999).

Comparing our findings with earlier studies is complicated by the fact that different studies use different criterion measures to operationalize disruptive behavior. Heilbrun et al. (1998), for example, rated only two types of aggression: (1) verbal aggression (shouting, threatening) and (2) physical aggression (pushing or hitting). They reported that PCL scores were predictive of verbal aggression but contrary to our findings, the PCL total score was also significantly correlated with physical aggression. In the present study, verbal aggression was divided into verbal abuse and verbal threats, and the category violation of hospital rules was included. In our opinion, this provides a more comprehensive picture of the nature and extent of incidents in a forensic hospital. Of interest is that although higher PCL-R Factor 1 scores were significantly associated with more verbal threat and total number of incidents, no such relationships were observed with verbal abuse and violation of hospital rules, whereas Factor 2 scores were significantly related to all incidents categories, except physical violence (i.e., verbal abuse, verbal threat, violation of rules, and total number of incidents).

All in all, given the relatively limited research that has been conducted on the institutional adjustment of Dutch forensic psychiatric patients, these findings are important in that they indicate that certain psychopathic traits (e.g., impulsivity, need for stimulation/proneness to boredom, poor behavioral controls) are associated with institutional misbehavior. Administering the PCL-R at admission may enable hospital staff to make appropriate initial placements with respect to treatment needs as well as disruptive potential. PCL-R psychopaths undermine the treatment milieu, specifically through verbal aggression and violation of hospital rules. The treatment and management of this patient group should be particularly focused on their impulsivity, lack of behavioral control and sensation seeking tendency. A highly structured treatment regime, possibly supported by the use of medication (e.g., SSRI's, low dose antipsychotics, Ritalin) should help reduce these characteristics, which is a prerequisite for further cognitive behavioral interventions, aimed at altering cognitive distortions, procriminal attitudes, lack of responsibility etc. (Serin & Kuriyichuk, 1994).

Chapter 6

PSYCHOPATHY AND CHANGE IN
DYNAMIC RISK FACTORS DURING
INPATIENT FORENSIC PSYCHIATRIC TREATMENT[1]

[1] Submitted for publication as:
Hildebrand, M., Ruiter, C. de , & Zaane, B. van *PCL-R Psychopathy and change in dynamic risk factors during inpatient forensic psychiatric treatment.*
We appreciate the input of the psychologists who, in addition to the first and second author, participated as assessors/raters. We also wish to thank the group leaders who completed T1 and T2 ICL-R assessments.

## SUMMARY

The main objective of the present study was to investigate the impact of treatment on forensic psychiatric patients, with a special emphasis on changes in dynamic risk factors for violence (e.g., impulse control, anger/hostility), and to relate these potential changes to psychopathy assessed with the Hare Psychopathy Checklist-Revised (PCL-R; Hare, 1991). In addition, we examined the relationship between psychopathy and treatment compliance, as indicated by the attendance rate of therapeutic activities. Eighty-seven male mentally disordered offenders were administered a standardized psychological assessment battery (semi-structured interviews, self-report inventories, performance-based personality test) upon admission (T1) and after two years of treatment (T2). Results indicated that the total sample showed limited change on indicators of dynamic risk factors, using different types of assessment techniques. Upon admission, psychopathy (PCL-R score $\geq$ 26) was significantly related to a limited number of indicators of dynamic risk upon admission. Contrary to our hypothesis, psychopathy was not significantly related to change scores on any of the indicators of dynamic risk. However, psychopaths showed the expected pattern of treatment noncompliance, compared to nonpsychopaths. The clinical and forensic implications of these findings are discussed.

## INTRODUCTION

Andrews et al. (1990; see also Andrews & Bonta, 2003; Andrews, Bonta, & Hoge, 1990) cogently argue that effective treatment to reduce recidivism requires the targeting of appropriate risk factors in offenders, including mentally disordered and/or psychopathic offenders. Drawn from the risk/need/responsivity theory (Andrews et al., 1990), the essence of the risk principle is that treatment is most effective when delivered proportionally to the level of risk of the patient. Thus, higher risk cases should receive more intensive service (i.e., multifaced intervention and of greater duration), whereas lower risk cases should receive less intervention. Risk level, moreover, is defined as the overall probability of criminal offending that is determined by both the number and severity of risk factors. The need principle refers to the (type of) treatment targets and suggests that interventions should be geared toward those factors that are most closely related to (the risk of) criminal offending (i.e., criminogenic needs). Examples of criminogenic need domains include problematic family and marital relationships, substance use/abuse, emotional or personal instability, and pro-criminal attitudes (Andrews & Bonta, 1994; Motiuk, 1995). The responsivity principle, finally, concerns the delivery of treatment programs in a style and mode that is consistent with the competence and learning style of the offender. The responsivity principle emphasizes the importance of patient characteristics and conditions that promote or impede positive change. By identifying personality and cognitive styles, treatment can be better tailored to the individual patient.

Two recently developed typologies of risk factors are of considerable utility. First, Hanson (1998; see also Andrews & Bonta, 2003) identified two general types of risk factors: *static* predictors and *dynamic* predictors. Static risk factors are those that are shown to be statistically related to recidivism and unable to change through intervention, and hence, can not be considered promising targets for treatment. Dynamic risk factors (criminogenic needs in Andrews and Bonta's terminology), on the other hand, are characteristics statistically related to recidivism that can (in principal) change, and when changed, are expected to result in a decrease in recidivism (Monahan & Appelbaum, 2000). Dynamic risk factors can be further subdivided into *stable* and *acute* dynamic risk factors (Hanson & Harris, 2000). Stable dynamic risk factors are expected to remain unchanged for months or years, whereas acute dynamic factors change very rapidly. Recent meta-analyses of the offender recidivism literature (Bonta, Law, & Hanson, 1998; Gendreau, Little, & Goggin, 1996) clearly revealed that dynamic 'need' variables correlate both with general and violent recidivism as well as or better than static factors that traditionally have been the focus of most research.

A second typology, designed by Kraemer et al. (1997) proposes a set of terms and definitions that incorporate the distinction between static and dynamic predictors, reflecting the current state of knowledge about such predictors. A fixed risk marker is one that can not be demonstrated to change, while a variable marker is a risk factor for which there is evidence to show it can change within an individual, either spontaneously or as a result of intervention. A further distinction can be drawn between variable and causal risk factors. Variable markers are those for which changes following intervention have not (yet) been shown to correspond with changes in risk, while causal markers are those that can be changed as a result of a deliberate intervention, and for which the change has been shown to correspond with a change in risk.

### Psychopathy, Treatment Involvement and Progress

Concerns about the effectiveness of treatment of forensic psychiatric patients focus particularly on patients with the diagnosis of psychopathic personality disorder. Psychopathic offenders present a major challenge to treatment providers because of the complex nature of the disorder itself, its co-morbidity with other types of mental disorder (e.g., Hart & Hare, 1989; Hildebrand & de Ruiter, 2004), and its association with other criminogenic risks and needs, such as substance abuse.

Given the compelling evidence for its validity, the Hare Psychopathy Checklist-Revised (Hare, 1991), a 20-item clinical rating scale, has emerged as the standard for the assessment of psychopathy. At least initially, PCL-R items were considered to be underpinned by two distinct but correlated factors: The "selfish, callous, and remorseless use of others" factor reflects the affective and interpersonal aspects of the disorder, whereas the behavioral items coalesce to form the "chronically, unstable and antisocial lifestyle; social deviance" factor (Hare, 1991, p. 76). Recently, Cooke and Michie (2001) concluded, on the basis of extensive cross-cultural research, that the two-factor model could not be supported. Using confirmatory factor analysis, they developed a hierarchical three-factor model, with distinct interpersonal, affective, and behavioral factors, uncontaminated by items reflecting criminal behavior. According to this three-factor model, criminality is seen as a possible consequence of psychopathy, as defined by its interpersonal, emotional and behavioral components. The PCL-R total score can range from 0 to 40; scores of 30 or higher are considered the criterion for psychopathy, although many scholars have recognized the value of different cut-off points in particular settings and populations (e.g., Cooke, 1995; Grann, Långström, Tengström, & Stålenheim, 1998; Harris, Rice, & Cormier, 1991).

On the basis of previous research investigating the relationship between psychopathy according to the PCL-R and response to treatment, four general conclusions can be drawn. First, psychopathic offenders engage in more disruptive behavior during treatment when compared to nonpsychopathic offenders (Gacono, Meloy, Sheppard, Speth, & Roske, 1995; Hare, Clarke, Grann, & Thornton, 2000; Heilbrun et al., 1998; Hildebrand, de Ruiter, & Nijman, 2004; Hill, Rogers, & Bickford, 1996; Rice, Harris, & Cormier, 1992). Rice et al. (1992), for example, reported that psychopathic offenders received more placements in seclusion for violent or disruptive behavior, more negative entries in the clinical records for disruptive or counter-therapeutic behavior, and more referrals to an institutional disciplinary sub-program than nonpsychopathic offenders.

Second, psychopathic offenders appear to be less likely to remain in treatment compared to nonpsychopathic offenders (e.g., Alterman, Rutherford, Cacciola, McKay, & Boardman, 1997; Ogloff, Wong, & Greenwood, 1990; Seto & Barbaree, 1999). For example, Ogloff et al. (1990) examined 80 adult male offenders who volunteered to attend a corrections-based therapeutic community (TC) program. It was found that the length of stay in the program was significantly shorter for psychopathic offenders ($n = 21$) than for other offenders ($n = 59$), mainly because they were more likely to be discharged from the program due to misbehavior or lack of motivation. Alterman et al. (1997) found that PCL-R scores were associated with uncompleted treatment. Hare et al. (2000) found that (PCL-R) psychopaths were less likely than nonpsychopaths to complete vocational and educational programs and were more likely than nonpsychopathic offenders to be fired from a prison job.

Third, several studies found that higher PCL-R scores are associated with lower scores on global measures of change (e.g., Hobson, Shine, & Roberts, 2000; Hughes, Hogue, Hollin, & Champion, 1997; Ogloff et al., 1990). For example, Hughes et al. (1997) found that higher PCL-R scores were associated with lower scores on a global measure of clinical change, primarily rated from in-therapy progress information provided by treatment staff. Ogloff et al. (1990) reported that patients in the high-psychopathy group received lower ratings by treatment staff (blind to PCL-R scores) on improvement than nonpsychopathic offenders.

Finally, the effectiveness of certain types of treatment in reducing (violent) re-offending among PCL-R psychopaths is questionable, and some treatments may even have iatrogenic effects (e.g., Hobson et al., 2000; Rice et al., 1992; Seto & Barbaree, 1999). Rice et al. (1992), for example, conducted a retrospective evaluation of a TC in a maximum-security institution for mentally disordered offenders, matching TC subjects with assessment-only subjects. Follow-up at a mean of 10.5 years after discharge showed that TC subjects with a PCL-R score ≥ 25 showed higher rates of recidivism, particularly violent recidivism, than a comparable *no-treatment control* group, suggesting that this particular type of treatment may have had an adverse impact on psychopathic offenders. Although considered innovative at the time, the TC treatment would not be considered appropriate according to the current research literature on "what works" with offenders (Andrews & Bonta, 1994; Cooke & Philip, 2001).

It can be concluded from the research cited above that, compared to nonpsychopaths, psychopathic offenders, place a significant burden on any treatment setting; PCL-R psychopathy is associated with higher levels of: (1) institutional misbehavior, (2) premature termination of treatment, and (3) post-treatment re-offending. However, there seems to be consensus among scholars that this does not warrant the conclusion that the disorder is immutable (Blackburn, 2001; Hare, 1998a; Hemphill & Hart, 2002; Lösel, 1998; Salekin, 2002; Wong, 2000). Most treatment studies are hampered by serious methodological problems and provide little guidance concerning what is or is not effective (e.g., Blackburn, 1993; Hart & Hare, 1997; Hemphill & Hart, 2002; Lösel, 1998; Wong, 2000). Major methodological weaknesses include the use of relatively small sample sizes; lack of (adequate) control groups; inadequate and limited outcome assessment; brief follow-up periods; failure to control for heterogeneity within treatment groups; failure to distinguish between treatments that target psychopathy versus those that treat psychopathy as a responsivity factor; inadequate description and implementation of treatment programs. But most of all, the lack of a treatment protocol specifically designed to address the criminogenic risk and needs exhibited by psychopaths.

## THE PRESENT STUDY

The main objective of the present study is to measure treatment progress in a sample of Dutch male offenders involuntarily admitted to a forensic psychiatric hospital, by change in dynamic risk factors as treatment outcome criterion. To the best of our knowledge, no study has been published before that systematically examined the association between PCL-R psychopathy and change in psychological measures of dynamic risk factors relevant to reoffending during treatment among forensic psychiatric patients. A dynamic risk factor, for the purpose of this study, is defined as a variable that relates to violence, may fluctuate with time and circumstances, and can be changed as a result of deliberate intervention (Webster, Douglas, Belfrage, & Link, 2000). The logic is as follows: Dynamic risk factors relate to actual violence; these dynamic factors are capable of indexing change; therefore, (systematic) change as measured by these factors is expected to be associated with violence risk reduction. We examined potential change in the following risk factors: Anger, egocentrism/narcissism, impulsivity, lack of insight, negative attitudes, and stress tolerance. These variables, while not exhaustive, cover a broad range of dynamic risk factors generally considered relevant to violent reoffending (e.g., Andrews & Bonta, 1994; Blackburn, 1998b; Bonta et al., 1998; Gendreau et al., 1996; Kay, Wolkenfeld, & Murrill, 1988; Megargee, 1976; Menzies, & Webster, 1995; Rice, Harris, Quinsey, & Cyr, 1990; Zamble & Quinsey, 1997; see also Douglas, Webster, Hart, Eaves, & Ogloff, 2001), and, at least in theory, are apt to change. We hypothesized that:

(1)    Upon admission to the hospital, offenders identified as psychopathic would show more pathology on indicators of dynamic risk than nonpsychopathic offenders;

(2)     psychopathic offenders would show more limited improvement after two years of
        inpatient treatment than nonpsychopathic offenders on outcome criteria. (It should
        be noted that, in the present study, psychopathy is considered as a responsivity
        factor).

An additional objective of this study is to investigate the relationship between
psychopathy and objective measures of treatment compliance, i.e., the extent to which the
patient actually participates in the assigned treatment program. It was hypothesized that
psychopathy is significantly related to a lower level of involvement on indicators of
treatment compliance, including the ratio of the number of attended to planned (individual)
psychotherapy sessions, attendance at work, educational activities, creative arts, and sports.

## METHOD

### SETTING

The study was conducted at the Dr. Henri van der Hoeven Kliniek, located in
Utrecht, the Netherlands, a 135-bed forensic psychiatric hospital for the treatment of
mentally disordered offenders who have been sentenced by criminal court to involuntary
commitment because of (severely) diminished responsibility for the offense(s) they
committed. In terms of legal status, most patients are sentenced to a 'maatregel van
terbeschikkingstelling' (TBS-order), a judicial measure which can be translated as
'disposal to be treated on behalf of the state'. The purpose of the TBS-order is to protect
society from offenders with unacceptably high risks of recidivism, directly through
involuntary admission to a secure forensic psychiatric hospital, and indirectly through the
treatment provided there. Every one or two years the court re-evaluates the patient in order
to determine whether the risk of (violent) recidivism is still too high and treatment needs to
be continued.

### TREATMENT MODEL

The hospital as a whole is organized as a therapeutic community. The general
treatment aim is a reduction in future violence risk by means of a positive change in those

risk factors that are associated with (sexual) violence and/or protective factors that are expected to buffer the effect of risk factors for the individual patient. A central concept in the treatment ideology of the hospital is the stimulation of the patient's awareness that he is responsible for his own life, including his offenses and his progress in treatment. Patients reside in living groups of around 10 patients, where they can develop and practice new (interpersonal) styles and skills. An adequately functioning outside social network is considered important to support the patient during treatment and during his reintegration into society. Treatment progress is evaluated every three months by the treatment team, which includes the supervising psychologist, group leaders, the psychotherapist and the social worker of the patient.

The treatment model is eclectic. A treatment program is offered, composed of individual and/or group therapy; job training, education, creative arts, and sports. Patients participate in group therapy programs, such as social skills training, aggression management, and substance abuse treatment. There are special group programs for pedophilic and adult-victim sexual offenders. Almost all patients receive individual cognitive-behavioral psychotherapy, with an emphasis on diminishing violence risk through interventions aimed at increasing the patient's insight and control over his behavior. The cognitive-behavioral therapy integrates several approaches, such as Young's (1994) schema-focused therapy for personality disorders, Linehan's (1993) dialectical behavior therapy and the offense script and relapse prevention method (Laws, 1989).

**SUBJECTS**

Subjects were 87 male forensic psychiatric patients admitted to the hospital between January 1, 1996 and May 31, 2001, who consented to administration of the baseline (T1) and follow-up (T2) assessments. The sample represents approximately 70% of available male subjects admitted to the hospital in the above-mentioned period. The remainder were either not examined or provided incomplete data (e.g., no T1 or T2 data), as a result of refusal of an interview, early referral to another facility, or severe clinical symptoms. The mean length of time between baseline assessment (T1) and retest (T2) was 21 months ($SD = 4$ months).

Mean age at admission was 30.1 years ($SD$ = 7 years; range = 19 to 47). Most (77%) of the men were White, and the others were of Surinamese / Antillean (14%), Mediterranean (7%) or other descent (2%). Sixty patients (69%) had never been married nor lived in a common law marriage. Forty-eight percent of the sample was convicted for (attempted) murder/homicide, and 25% for sexual offences (i.e., sexual assault, rape, child molest); the others for (aggravated) assault, robbery with violence, threat, and arson.

**ASSESSMENTS**

In order to obtain insight into factors related to the patient's (sexual) violence risk and to develop an individual case formulation that provides a basis treatment plan and for monitoring the patient's progress during treatment, all patients are administered a standardized battery of psychological evaluation instruments upon admission (T1), including semi-structured interviews, self-report inventories and performance-based personality tests. *Multimethod* assessments are employed, because distinct assessment methods provide unique sources of data. On the basis of a large array of evidence, Meyer et al. (2000; see also Meyer, 1997) argue that "optimal knowledge in clinical practice (as in research) is obtained from the sophisticated integration of information derived from a multimethod assessment battery" (p. 155). Multimethod assessment is particularly important in forensic subjects, who tend to be more prone to defensive responding, faking good or faking bad than subjects who are not assessed under mandatory conditions. By using multiple methods to assess the same symptoms (e.g., impulsivity, egocentricity) the findings with one method can be cross validated against the findings obtained with another method.

In order to provide information on treatment progress, as many patients as possible are re-tested with the same assessment battery (interviews not included), 18-24 months after admission (T2). The 'what works' literature (e.g., Andrews et al., 1990) highlights the importance of having evaluation procedures built into programs to check they are meeting the stated objectives as part of a continuous review process. In addition, behavior change (the ultimate goal) is not expected to occur in a vacuum: concomitant changes in personality, beliefs, and attitudes are expected. All instruments were administered according to standard administration procedures explained in the respective test manuals.

*Semi-structured interviews*. Upon admission, patients were interviewed to obtain data on PCL-R psychopathy and on DSM-IV personality disorders. Psychopathy was assessed using the Dutch language version (Vertommen, Verheul, de Ruiter, & Hildebrand, 2002) of the PCL-R (Hare, 1991).[2] The standard procedure for scoring the PCL-R was employed in 77 cases. This entails coding on the basis of a semi-structured interview and extensive file information. Items were scored on a 3-point scale (0 = *item does not apply*, 1 = *item applies to a certain extent*, 2 = *item definitely applies*). PCL-R interviews were videotaped, for which patients had to give their written informed consent, and PCL-R ratings were made by (at least) two independent raters.[3] The remaining 10 cases were based on file information only (two independent raters). PCL-R consensus scores were used in all subsequent data-analyses.

DSM-IV Axis II diagnoses were obtained by administration of the Dutch translation of the Structured Interview for DSM-IV Disorders of Personality (SIDP-IV; Pfohl, Blum, & Zimmerman, 1994; de Jong, Derks, van Oel, & Rinne, 1996). Diagnostic criteria were rated after the interview was completed and the interviewer had also examined available file information. No interrater reliability data were collected for Axis II diagnoses, but in most cases the scoring was reviewed by a second, senior-level clinical psychologist, who also knew the patient.[4]

*Self-report inventories*. In addition to the interview methods, patients completed a number of self-report measures, including the Minnesota Multiphasic Personality Inventory-2 (MMPI-2; Butcher, Dahlstrom, Graham, Tellegen, & Kaemmer, 1989; Flemish/Dutch version: Sloore, Derksen, de Mey, & Hellenbosch, 1993), a 567-item (true/false) personality inventory that provides information on a subject's personality and psychopathology. In addition to the primary three validity scales and 10 clinical scales, the MMPI-2 includes (Harris-Lingoes) subscales that identify distinct components within the

---

[2] Thirty-four patients were administered the PCL-R interview at T2.
[3] Twenty-four patients refused to give consent for videotaping the interview; eight of them agreed with a joint interview approach (one rater conducted the interview while a second rater was present as an observer); six refused the presence of a second observer, and PCL-R scores had to be based on the judgment of a single interviewer (MH or CdR).
[4] Nine of the 87 patients were diagnosed using the Dutch translation (van den Brink & de Jong, 1992) of the Structured Interview for DSM-III-R (SIDP-R; Pfohl, Blum, Zimmerman, & Stangl, 1989). This is a consequence of the duration of the data collection, which started before the Dutch SIDP-IV became available.

more heterogeneous clinical scales as well as a series of supplementary and content scales that further identify more specific psychological symptoms.

The Dutch revised version of the Interpersonal Checklist (ICL; LaForge & Suczek, 1955; Dutch version: ICL-R; de Jong, van den Brink, & Jansma, 2000) is a 160-item self-report instrument designed to measure interpersonal style. Each item (rated present/absent) is assigned to one of 10 dimensions. Scores on each dimension can range from 0 to 16. Within each dimension, items are designed to range from adaptive manifestations of a particular interpersonal reflex to extreme and maladaptive manifestations. Scores between 4-12 are generally considered indicative of adaptive behavior. Dimensions are labeled *PA* (managerial-autocratic), *BC* (competitive-exploitive), *DE* (aggressive-blunt), *FG* (distrustful- skeptical), *nFnG* (reserved-aloof), *HI* (modest-self-effacing), *JK* (docile-dependent), *LM* (cooperative-overconventional), *NO* (responsible-overgenerous), and *nNnO* (extravert-gregarious). The scores on these dimensions can be transformed into a vector score, which roughly describes the interpersonal style in terms of the degree of power or control in an interaction (dominance versus submissiveness) and the degree of affiliation (hostility versus friendliness/nurturance).   To determine the degree of convergence between patient and observer ratings, as a general procedure in our hospital, the ICL-R is also completed by staff members (i.e., a consensus rating of at least two group leaders who interact with the patient on a daily basis).

The Barratt Impulsiveness Scale-11 (BIS-11; Barratt, 1994) is a 30-item self-report measure of impulsivity. Items are rated from 1 (rarely/never) to 4 (almost always/always). Barratt (1994) provided initial evidence for a three-factor structure of the BIS-11 in analyses using 151 college students: An ideomotor factor (*IM*, 12 items; acting without thinking); a careful planning dimension (*CAPL*, 5 items; attention to details), and a coping stability factor (*COST*, 8 items; lack of concern for the future).

The Novaco Anger Scale (NAS; Novaco, 1994)[5] consists of 73 items, which comprise two sections: Part A (48 items) focuses on anger reactions, and is divided into three domains (a cognitive, arousal, and behavioral domain), each domain having four subscales.

---

[5] BIS-11 and NAS translated with permission into Dutch by Cecile Vandeputte and Corine de Ruiter.

Responses are made on a three-point scale, ranging from 'never true' to 'always true'. Part B (25 items) is intended to measure anger intensity across a range of potentially provoking situations, and is divided into five subscales. Responses are made on a four-point scale, ranging from 'not angry' to 'very angry'. For both Part A and Part B holds that higher scores reflect more feelings or cognitions associated with anger.

*Performance-based personality test.* Patients were administered the Rorschach Inkblot Method (RIM; Rorschach, 1921/1942) using Exner's (2001) Comprehensive System (CS) scoring system. The RIM consists of the consecutive presentation of a set of 10 achromatic and chromatic inkblots published by Huber Verlag. The basic assumption underlying the Rorschach is that personality characteristics influence the response process that takes place after the examiner has presented each card and asked the subject "What might this be?" According to Exner (1993), the RIM is a problem-solving task, in which the stimulus features of the blots are just as relevant as the idiosyncratic projections of the subject. The administration and scoring of the Rorschach followed standardized procedures outlined by Exner (1993, 2001). All Rorschach protocols were scored by the administrator and rescored by a colleague. Consensus ratings were obtained, which were used in all subsequent analyses. Interrater reliability was examined using 52 protocols. Interscorer reliability measures were obtained for eight major categories of Rorschach CS variables, as recommended by Exner, Kinder, and Curtiss (1995).

The percentage of agreement between raters was as follows for each major category of Rorschach CS variables: Location and Developmental Quality = 92%; Determinants = 88%; Form Quality = 84%; Pairs = 95%; Contents = 94%; Populars = 97%; Organizational Activity (Z-score) = 92%, and Special Scores = 82%, indicating good to excellent interscorer reliability (Smid, 2003). In fact, for each category, agreement measures met the standards recommended by Exner et al. (1995).

## EXCLUSION CRITERIA

Prior to data analysis, all MMPI-2 test protocols were screened for inconsistent responding and protocol invalidity. MMPI-2s were considered valid if 30 or fewer items were omitted, True Response Inconsistency (TRIN) T-scores were < 80, and Variable Response Inconsistency (VRIN) T-scores were < 80. Using these exclusion criteria, three

MMPI-2 protocols were eliminated. In accordance with Exner's (1993) requirements, only Rorschach protocols with a number of ≥ 14 responses were included in the study. Using this exclusion criterion, protocols (either T1 and/or T2 ) of 19 patients had to be excluded from study.

RECORD REVIEWS

Lifetime Axis I diagnoses were established by the first author using all available data (e.g., earlier psychological and psychiatric reports, earlier diagnoses, current psychiatric or psychological assessments). No interrater reliability data were collected for Axis I diagnoses. However, for 76 patients (87%), diagnoses were reviewed by three independent raters (cf. Hildebrand & de Ruiter, 2004): a senior-diagnostician and a senior psychotherapist of the hospital staff, and the second author. Missing diagnoses were added and disagreements between the four raters were discussed and resolved, and a set of final consensus diagnoses for the 76 patients in the sample was established. This procedure (i.e., using consensus diagnoses) was chosen to maximize.

Furthermore, computerized hospital records were reviewed to provide information about treatment (non)compliance, number of missed and attended (individual) psychotherapy sessions, work and educational activities, creative arts, and sports.

INTERVIEWERS

All psychological assessments were conducted by a pool of 10 (research) psychologists with master's or doctoral degrees. All were experienced in assessment and/or treatment of (forensic) psychiatric patients (cf. Hildebrand & de Ruiter, 2004; Hildebrand et al., 2002). The psychologists ($n = 5$) who administered the RIM were trained in the CS.[6]

---

[6] One of them (Corine de Ruiter) is active as Rorschach instructor, and member of the faculty of Rorschach Workshops, Asheville, NC, USA.

## SELECTED INDICATORS OF DYNAMIC RISK FACTORS

Selected variables from the self-report inventories and the RIM that provide information on the dynamic (risk) factors (i.e., anger / hostility, egocentrism / narcissism, stress tolerance, impulsivity, lack of insight, and negative attitudes), were analyzed in order to examine change during forensic psychiatric treatment. For the RIM variables, each variable has a clinically significant cut-off score, above which the score is considered to be problematic;[7] all scores were dichotomized (0 = *normal*; 1 = *problematic*). The frequencies (percentage scores) of problematic scores on each of the RIM variables was assessed for psychopathic and nonpsychopathic patients. For the ICL-R, ratings of patient and observers (group leaders) were analyzed. Dynamic risk factors were selected because they have support in the scientific literature as risk markers of violence. The following variables were selected from self-report inventories and the RIM as indicators of dynamic risk factors:

### Anger/Hostility

*NAS*. Part A and Part B total scores were used as measures of anger.

*MMPI-2*. For the MMPI-2, selected variables were the Anger Content scale (*ANG*; 16 items), the Cynicism Content scale (*CYN*; 23 items), and the 28-item Overcontrolled-Hostility Supplementary scale (*O-H*; Megargee, Cook, & Mendelsohn, 1967). *ANG* is concerned with poorly controlled anger (Schill & Wang, 1990); *CYN* measures to what extent an individual distrusts others because they act only out of self-interest; the *O-H* scale is a hostility measure shown to be associated with aggressive and violent acts in correctional settings (Graham, 2000).

*ICL-R*. The *DE* scale score was chosen as an anger / hostility variable.

*RIM CS*. The variable *S > 3* was used to measure oppositionality / internalized anger.

### Negative Distrustful Attitudes

*MMPI-2*. Scale 6 (Paranoid, *Pa*; 40 items) taps externalizing processes, such as hypervigilance, and scanning for 'evidence' of hostile intentions or actions of others.

---

[7] Guidelines for interpreting RIM CS variables are given by Exner (1993, 2001) and Weiner (1998).

*ICL-R*. The *FG* scale score was chosen as indicator of distrustfulness.

**Egocentrism/Narcissism**

*MMPI-2*. Three MMPI-2 scales were chosen as indicators of egocentrism/narcissism: The 50-item Superlative Self-Presentation (*S*) scale, the Harris-Lingoes (H-L) Subscale Social Imperturbability (*Pd3*; 6 items), and the H-L Subscale Ego Inflation (*Ma4*; 9 items). The *S* scale assesses the tendency of some persons to unrealistically report positive attributes, and good adjustment (Butcher & Han, 1995); *Pd3* reflects a highly aggressive and insouciant sociability consistent with a desire to use interpersonal relationships to manipulate, intimidate, and exploit; *Ma4* measures the grandiosity typical of the (hypo)manic person. High scorers usually have unrealistic appraisals of their own abilities and self-worth, and become angry when one's importance is not appreciated.

*RIM CS*. $Fr + rF > 0$ (narcissistic-like tendencies); $3r + (2) / R > .43$ (unusual degree of self-preoccupation), and $PER > 3$ (overly defensive of one's self-image; argumentative) were selected as indicators of egocentrism/narcissism.

**Impulsivity**

*BIS-11*. Scores on *IM*, *CAPL*, and *COST*, and the BIS-11 total score were used as indicators of impulsivity.

*RIM CS*. Variables to measure impulsivity comprised: $CF + C > FC + 1$ (lack of emotional control) and $Zd < -3.0$ (inattention to detail; superficial scanning).

**Lack of Insight**

*ICL-R*. Perceived differences [patients scoring lower on 'negative' dimensions (i.e., *BC*, *DE*, *FG*) and higher on 'positive' dimensions (*nFnG*, *LM*, *NO*), compared to staff] between patient and staff ratings on selected ICL-R dimensions were considered indicators of lack of insight.

*RIM CS*. $FD = 0$ (lack of introspective capacities).

**Stress Tolerance**

*MMPI-2*. Stress tolerance was measured with the Ego Strength (*Es*; 52 items) Supplementary scale (Barron, 1953). High scoring subjects are independent, and self-reliant; they show flexibility and tolerance; at times they are outspoken and nonconforming toward authority; low scorers are unstable, overreactive, and subject to confusion in the face of stress.

*RIM CS.* Indices were $D < 0$ (a person's stress tolerance and capacity for control) and *adjusted D* $< 0$ (controls for certain situational stressors and is reflective of the respondent's common capacity to tolerate stress and control his behavior) scores.

## TREATMENT COMPLIANCE

In order to provide information on treatment (non)compliance, computerized hospital case files were reviewed for the number of missed and attended therapeutic activities. The attendance rate of (individual) psychotherapy sessions, work, educational activities, creative arts, and sports were considered indicators of treatment compliance.

## DATA ANALYSIS

Treatment outcome was investigated as the change relative to the baseline scores. Accordingly, it is not the absolute level of mental health that was taken as an indicator of success, but the degree of improvement. The factor of interest to be tested was the effect of psychopathy. To study the effect of PCL-R psychopathy on baseline assessment and treatment progress (change at T2 relative to baseline scores) independent *t*-tests were calculated. We tested each dynamic risk factor separately, resulting in Bonferroni adjusted (Stevens, 1986) Type 1 error rates varying from .007 (.05 / 7) for self-report indicators of Anger/hostility to .017 (.05 / 3) for self-report indicators of Negative Distrustful Attitudes and Egocentrism. For RIM CS variables, the chi-square statistic was used to determine differences between T1 and T2 scores, also with Bonferroni correction to reduce the risk of chance capitalization.

The relation between PCL-R scores and attendance rate of psychotherapy sessions, work, education, sports, and creative arts was evaluated with Pearson product-moment correlations, with $\alpha$ set at .05.

## RESULTS

### Diagnostic Status

#### PSYCHOPATHY

The mean (adjusted sum) total PCL-R score  for the total sample was 20.97 ($SD$ = 8.37), with a range from 3 to 38, a median score of 22 and a mode of 17. The kurtosis of the PCL-R total score was − .716 ($SE$ = .511). PCL-R scores were normally distributed (Kolmogorov-Smirnov $Z$ = .625, $p$ = .829). The mean Factor 1 score was 9.19 ($SD$ = 3.88), the mean Factor 2 score was 9.35 ($SD$ = 5.53). Twenty-seven patients (31%) were classified as 'psychopaths', using a cut-off of 26, which is often used in European research (e.g., Grann et al., 1998; Rasmussen et al., 1999). When a cut-off score of 30, as used by Hare (1991), was employed, 16 patients (18%) were classified as 'psychopaths'. Nine patients (10%) had a PCL-R score < 10.

#### DSM-IV AXIS I AND AXIS II DISORDERS

Thirteen patients (15%) met criteria for schizophrenia or another psychotic disorder. Forty-five patients (52%) met criteria for (at least) one substance related disorder (i.e., any alcohol or other substance related disorder).

The prevalence of personality disorders in the sample was high. Seventy-four patients (85%; valid data obtained for 86 patients) received at least one Axis II diagnosis. Co-morbidity on Axis II was common: of the 74 patients given a diagnosis, 38 (51%) received multiple diagnoses. The mean number of personality disorders per patient, for patients with at least one disorder was 1.85. As expected, most personality disorders were Cluster B disorders, followed by Cluster A. The most frequently diagnosed disorder was antisocial personality disorder ($n$ = 41), followed by narcissistic ($n$ = 23), borderline ($n$ = 19), and paranoid personality disorder ($n$ = 15).

## Indicators of Dynamic Risk

### BASELINE SCORES OF PSYCHOPATHIC AND NONPSYCHOPATHIC PATIENTS

Upon admision, only two indicators demonstrated significant (Bonferroni adjusted) differences between psychopathic and nonpsychopathic patients. Psychopathic patients had significantly higher scores on the 'Anger / Hostility' indicator *ICL-R DE* (for patient ratings, $t = -2.96$, $p = .004$; for staff ratings, $t = -2.91$, $p = .005$), compared to nonpsychopaths, indicating higher levels of anger. Table 1 summarizes the mean baseline scores for all indicators of dynamic risk factors for psychopathic and nonpsychopathic patients.

TABLE 1

*Psychopathy in Relation to Baseline Assessment (T1) of Dynamic Risk Factors and Differences in Change Scores from Baseline to Retest (T2)*

| Outcome Criteria | $df^b$ | Baseline Assessment | | | | Difference in Change Scores[a] |
|---|---|---|---|---|---|---|
| | | PCL-R < 26 M (SD) | | PCL-R ≥ 26 M (SD) | | t or $\chi^2$ (RIM) | t or $\chi^2$ (RIM) |
| **Anger** | | | | | | | |
| *Novaco* | | | | | | | |
| Part A | 63 | 79.9 | (12.6) | 86.1 | (12.0) | -1.94 | -0.54 |
| Part B | 63 | 50.9 | (11.7) | 50.3 | (11.6) | 0.20 | -0.87 |
| *MMPI-2* | | | | | | | |
| ANG | 82 | 51.1 | (12.7) | 57.3 | (13.7) | -2.04 | 0.46 |
| CYN | 82 | 47.3 | (11.7) | 52.6 | (13.2) | -1.83 | -0.11 |
| O-H | 82 | 60.0 | (12.3) | 61.2 | (11.6) | -0.44 | -0.08 |
| *ICL-R* | | | | | | | |
| DE (patient) | 85 | 7.3 | ( 2.4) | 8.8 | ( 2.0) | **-2.96**[*] | -1.03 |
| DE (staff) | 64 | 5.5 | ( 2.8) | 7.7 | ( 3.2) | **-2.91**[*] | -1.84 |
| *RIM* | | | | | | | |
| S > 3 | 58 | T1 25% | T2 30% | T1 36% | T2 43% | 0.61 | 0.85 |
| **Negative attitudes** | | | | | | | |
| *MMPI-2* | | | | | | | |
| Scale 6 (Pa) | 82 | 62.9 | (11.1) | 59.8 | (10.8) | 1.20 | 0.77 |
| *ICL-R* | | | | | | | |
| FG (patient) | 85 | 6.8 | ( 2.7) | 8.1 | ( 2.9) | -1.99 | -0.64 |
| FG (staff) | 64 | 9.2 | ( 3.3) | 11.1 | ( 2.7) | -2.35 | -1.45 |
| **Egocentrism** | | | | | | | |
| *MMPI-2* | | | | | | | |
| S | 82 | 50.6 | (11.8) | 45.4 | (13.2) | 1.82 | -0.01 |
| Pd3 | 82 | 49.6 | (11.0) | 53.8 | (7.8) | -1.75 | -0.69 |
| Ma4 | 82 | 52.5 | (10.6) | 55.6 | (11.6) | -1.19 | 0.28 |
| *RIM* | | | | | | | |
| Fr+rF > 0 | 58 | T1 25% | T2 30% | T1 29% | T2 29% | 0.07 | 0.01 |
| 3R+(2)/R>.43 | 58 | T1 30% | T2 27% | T1 36% | T2 43% | 0.19 | 1.21 |
| PER > 3 | 58 | T1 16% | T2 5% | T1 14% | T2 21% | 0.02 | 3.84 |

*(table continues)*

**TABLE 1** (*cont.*)

| Outcome Criteria | $df^b$ | Baseline Assessment PCL-R < 26 M (SD) | | Baseline Assessment PCL-R ≥ 26 M (SD) | | $t/\chi^{2c}$ | Difference in Change Scores[a] $t/\chi^{2c}$ |
|---|---|---|---|---|---|---|---|
| **Impulsivity** | | | | | | | |
| *Barratt* | | | | | | | |
| IM | 63 | 24.2 | (4.6) | 25.4 | (3.5) | -1.16 | 1.41 |
| CAPL | 63 | 10.1 | (2.2) | 11.2 | (2.6) | -1.87 | -0.23 |
| COST | 63 | 15.7 | (2.9) | 15.9 | (3.0) | -0.20 | 0.21 |
| Total | 63 | 60.3 | (8.9) | 63.0 | (7.2) | -1.25 | 0.40 |
| | | | | | | | |
| *RIM* | | | | | | | |
| CF+C>FC+1 | 58 | T1 36% | T2 39% | T1 21% | T2 29% | 1.08 | 0.47 |
| Zd < -3.0 | 58 | T1 32% | T2 30% | T1 14% | T2 21% | 1.63 | 0.35 |
| | | | | | | | |
| **Lack of insight**[c,d] | | | | | | | |
| *ICL-R* | | | | | | | |
| BC | 69 | -0.1 | (3.9) | 0.7 | (3.7) | -0.81 | -0.09 |
| DE | 69 | 2.0 | (2.9) | 1.1 | (3.1) | 1.21 | 1.31 |
| FG | 69 | -2.2 | (3.9) | -3.1 | (3.5) | 0.90 | 0.65 |
| nFnG | 69 | -0.9 | (3.9) | 0.9 | (3.5) | -1.81 | -1.52 |
| LM | 69 | 2.6 | (3.4) | 4.5 | (2.2) | -2.45 | -1.91 |
| NO | 69 | 5.2 | (3.7) | 6.5 | (3.1) | -1.51 | 0.21 |
| | | | | | | | |
| *RIM* | | | | | | | |
| FD = 0 | 58 | T1 52% | T2 61% | T1 50% | T2 43% | 0.02 | 1.48 |
| | | | | | | | |
| **Stress tolerance** | | | | | | | |
| *MMPI-2* Es | 82 | 43.6 | (12.9) | 44.4 | (14.4) | -0.25 | -0.41 |
| | | | | | | | |
| *RIM* | | | | | | | |
| D < 0 | 58 | T1 46% | T2 50% | T1 36% | T2 50% | 0.41 | 0.00 |
| adjusted D<0 | 58 | T1 30% | T2 23% | T1 21% | T2 43% | 0.35 | 2.15 |

*Note.* MMPI-2=Minnesota Multiphasic Personality Inventory; ANG=Anger scale; CYN=Cynicism scale; O-H = Overcontrolled-Hostility scale; Pa=Paranoia scale; S=Superlative Self-Presentation scale; Pd3=Harris-Lingoes scale Social Imperturbability; Ma4=Harris-Lingoes scale Ego Inflation; Es=Ego Strength scale; ICL-R=Interpersonal Checklist-Revised; BC=competitive-exploitive; DE=aggressive-blunt; FG=skeptical-distrustful; nFnG=reserved-aloof; LM=cooperative-overconventional; NO=responsible-overgenerous; RIM=Rorschach Inkblot Method. IM=ideo-motor; CAPL=careful planning; COST=coping stability. [a]Except for Rorschach variables, T2 scores are change scores indicating the degree of progress in relation to baseline scores. [b]Due to missing data not all numbers add up to equal the total sample. [c]Scores are mean differences between patient and staff ratings. [d]df for T2 = 64.
*$p$ < .01. Significant (Bonferroni adjusted) values are in bold.

**Degree of Improvement**

*Total sample*. The overall finding over the course of treatment indicates that for the sample *as a whole* there were only few scales (4 of 33) demonstrating significant change between T1 and T2. With regard to the 'Anger / hostility' indicators, *t*-tests revealed that the *total sample* became less cynical on *MMPI-2 Cyn* [T1: $M = 49.0$, T2: $M = 45.9$; $t$ (1,83) $= 2.89$, $p = .005$], and more dominant and assertive on ICL-R *DE*, according to staff ratings [T1: $M = 6.2$, T2: $M = 7.3$; $t$ (1,66) $= -2.89$, $p = .005$]. Also, patients became more extravert on the 'Egocentrism' indicator *MMPI-2 Pd3* [T1: $M = 50.9$, T2: $M = 53.3$; $t$ (1,83) $= -2.49$, $p = .015$]. Interestingly, staff ratings on the 'Negative Attitude' indicator *ICL-R FG* were significantly higher at T2 [T1: $M = 9.7$, T2: $M = 11.1$; $t$ (1,65) $= -3.00$, $p = .004$].

*Psychopathic versus nonpsychopathic patients*. Psychopathy was *not* related in any way to treatment progress as indicated by change relative to the baseline scores (see Table 1).

**Psychopathy and Treatment Compliance**

The correlations between PCL-R scores and attendance rates of different therapeutic activities are displayed in Table 2. PCL-R total ($r = -.34$, $p < .001$) and Factor 2 (work: $r = -.34$, $p < .001$; education: $r = -.34$, $p < .001$) scores were negatively associated with attendance of work and education; the higher the PCL-R total and Factor 2 score the worse was the patient's attendance rate. Attendance of individual psychotherapy sessions, sports, and creative arts, was not related to PCL-R scores. Factor 1 was not in any way related to treatment compliance.

TABLE 2
*Correlations Between Psychopathy and Attendance Rate of Therapeutic Activities*

| | PCL-R | | |
|---|---|---|---|
| **Therapeutic Activities** | Total score | Factor 1 | Factor 2 |
| Psychotherapy ($n = 84$) | .15 | .19 | .15 |
| Work ($n = 86$) | **-.34**$^{**}$ | -.17 | **-.34**$^{**}$ |
| Education ($n = 86$) | **-.34**$^{**}$ | -.13 | **-.30**$^{*}$ |
| Sports ($n = 86$) | -.11 | -.02 | -.05 |
| Creative arts ($n = 84$) | -.14 | -.02 | -.07 |

*Note.* PCL-R = Psychopathy Checklist-Revised. Significant correlations are in bold.
$^{*}p < .01$. $^{**}p \leq .001$ (all two-tailed).

## Comparison Between Patients Included in the Sample and
## Patients Tested Only Upon Admission

Due to various reasons (e.g., refusal, referral to another facility), 28 patients were tested only at T1 and were therefore excluded from the present study. It is relevant whether psychopathy scores and scores on dynamic risk factors for these patients were different from patients who provided a complete data set. If so, there could be a selection bias. Comparisons between patients who did and who did not provide a complete data set, indicated that the PCL-R total score of the dropouts  was significantly higher than the mean PCL-R score of those who provided a T1 and a T2 [$M = 24.9$ versus $M = 21.0$; $t (1, 107) = 2.02$, $p = .046$]. There were no differences, however, in the presence or absence of categorical psychopathy, $\chi^2 (1, 114) = 1.65$, $p = .199$. With regard to the outcome criteria, $t$-tests revealed that the drop-outs were significantly more cynical [$CYN$: $t (1,113) = 2.16$, $p = .033$] and less egocentric on $S$ [$t (1,113) = -2.12$, $p = .036$] and $Ma4$ [$t (1,113) = 2.49$, $p = .014$] compared to patients who provided a complete data set.

## DISCUSSION

The purpose of the present study was to explore the extent to which change in specific psychological measures of dynamic risk factors relevant to reoffending could differentiate between psychopathic and nonpsychopathic patients during inpatient forensic psychiatric treatment. It was hypothesized that upon admission to the hospital, psychopathic offenders would show higher levels of disturbance on indicators of dynamic risk than nonpsychopathic offenders. We expected psychopaths to show more limited improvement after two years of treatment than nonpsychopathic patients. In addition, this study investigated the relationship between psychopathy and treatment compliance, as indicated by the attendance rates of different kinds of therapeutic activities. We expected treatment noncompliance to be more characteristic for patients with high PCL-R scores.

Three major findings are evident from our treatment outcome study. First, dividing patients according to presence or absence of psychopathy revealed that, at baseline assessment, psychopathic patients showed only significantly higher levels of disturbance on two indicators of the dynamic risk factor 'Anger/hostility'. Thus, our first hypothesis was not confirmed. Contrary to our expectation, psychopaths and nonpsychopaths showed more similarities than differences in dynamic risk factors.

Second, the sample *as a whole* did not improve on most of the indicators of dynamic risk. Contrary to our second hypothesis, no differential treatment response was found between psychopathic and nonpsychopathic patients.

Third, our results provide partial support for the association between psychopathy and treatment compliance, i.e., the extent to which the patient actually participates in the assigned treatment program. High PCL-R total and Factor 2 scores were significantly related to a lower level of involvement in education and work, suggesting that psychopathic patients tend to put less effort into the treatment program. It is noteworthy that psychopathic patients show similar attendance to activities such as sports and creative arts, the 'fun' activities.

One can speculate about why changes in dynamic risk factors were nonexistent during the two-year treatment course. Two explanations arise from the study. A first explanation for our findings is that the patients in our sample have such severe psychopathology, which is very difficult to change; the second concerns the type of treatment program offered at the hospital.

With regard of the first explanation, it should be mentioned that our sample consisted only of high risk mentally disordered offenders. Changes in dynamic risk factors such as anger, egocentrism, impulsivity, lack of insight, and stress tolerance may very well be very hard to accomplish. To illustrate this point, Belfrage and Douglas (2002) examined change in violence risk factors in forensic psychiatric patients across multiple assessment periods, using the HCR-20. They found that, in a sub-sample of 70 high risk patients undergoing long-term treatment, HCR-20 dynamic risk factors changed only modestly. Also, the lack of change on indicators of dynamic risk could be due to the limited time period between T1 and T2 (i.e., two years of treatment). Possibly, patients improve on indicators of dynamic risk factors at a slower pace. Most patients in our sample will continue treatment for an extended period and future assessments (after four years of treatment) may reveal the hypothesized changes.

The second possible explanation for our findings is that it may be that the treatment program provided at the hospital deserves review or alteration. Although the program takes into account that patients present a diversity of (behavior) problems, it is largely based on the principles of the therapeutic community: An environment is created in which complex interpersonal and community processes become central therapeutic factors (e.g., Dolan, 1998). Previous research indicates that milieu therapies permit psychopathic patients to con staff into believing they are making progress (Hare et al., 2000; Hobson et al, 2000). The treatment program provided in our hospital is *not* specifically designed to *systematically* change the dynamic risk factors we studied. Alteration of the treatment program into a program based on the principles of risk, need and responsivity, focusing on reducing the risk of violence and destructiveness by modifying the cognitions and behaviors that directly precipitate violent behavior, may maximize change. It may also be that the standard of service delivery could be increased by forming homogenous groups of patients allowing the development of specialized wards to target the needs of different groups of patients (Müller-Isberner, 1993; Rice, Harris, Quinsey, & Cyr, 1990), with the specificity of each ward being based on both patient's treatment needs and security requirements. As a standard procedure, criminogenic needs identified during baseline assessment should become treatment targets, and for each an explicit treatment plan needs to specify how change is to be accomplished. Appropriate interventions delivered in this manner may produce favorable results in the treatment of this high risk group of offenders.

Our results provide support for the negative association between psychopathy and treatment compliance, as high PCL-R total and Factor 2 scores were significantly related to a lower level of involvement in education and work, suggesting that psychopathic patients tend to put less effort into the treatment program. Attendance rates of individual psychotherapy, sports and creative arts, however, were not related to PCL-R scores. In general, these findings are in line with earlier findings (e.g., Ogloff et al., 1990; Hobson et al., 2000) supporting the value of the PCL-R as a significant correlate of treatment compliance in forensic inpatients. Hobson et al. (2000), for example, found that the PCL-R total and Factor 1 score were associated with negative behaviors shown in therapy groups. They also reported significant correlations between PCL-R scores (total and factor scores) and wing behavior. Off wing activities (e.g., education, charity work) were inversely related to Factor 2 scores. Contrary to the research of Hobson et al. (2000), who found evidence that attention should be given equally to Factor 1 and Factor 2 scores, the present research indicates that Factor 2 is of particular importance in forecasting and effectively managing treatment compliance. In the present study, the Factor 1 score was in no way associated with treatment compliance. It should be noted though that comparing our findings with earlier studies is complicated by the fact that different studies use different criterion measures to operationalize treatment compliance. For example, Hobson et al. (2000) used an officer-completed behavior checklist to monitor institutional adjustment, whereas in the present study computerized hospital records were reviewed to provide information about the level of involvement in therapeutic activities.

A number of limitations of this study should be noted. The first, and perhaps the most significant, limitation is the lack of an adequate control group. We did not use a true experimental design, one in which treatment and control groups were performed prior to treatment using random assignment and in which group equivalence with respect to theoretically important variables was evaluated (e.g., Hemphill & Hart, 2002). Placement in our hospital followed specific criteria, and an equivalent control group could not be formed for legal and therapeutic reasons.

Second, data collection was restricted to one forensic psychiatric hospital. The extent to which these treatment outcome findings apply to the treatment programs offered in other (Dutch) forensic psychiatric hospitals is not known. The level of success may be different for other hospitals, which offer different programs. It should also be considered whether lack of power is a main reason for the non-significant findings. Generally, lack of power may occur when the sample size is small and when the base rate of psychopathy is low. In the present study, 27 patients (31%) were diagnosed as psychopathic (PCL-R $\geq$ 26), and there were not even trends in the direction of the hypothesis that psychopathic patients show more limited improvement after two years of inpatient treatment than nonpsychopathic offenders. Therefore, a larger sample size is not likely to change the present results.

Another limitation is the lack of reliable and clinically meaningful measures that can be applied to evaluate a complex treatment regime, such as the one in our hospital (Hughes, Hogue, Hollin, & Champion, 1997). It may be that the measures we employed were not sensitive enough to evaluate change in dynamic risk variables over time. However, the notable stability of Rorschach indicators in this study contrasts with earlier treatment outcome studies which found positive changes on (many of) these indicators (Abraham et al., 1994; Exner & Andronikof-Sanglade, 1992; Weiner & Exner, 1991). Weiner and Exner (1991), for example, used 27 RIM CS indicators of adjustment difficulty to evaluate treatment effects in a sample of (nonforensic) outpatients, mainly suffering from anxiety disorders or depression. They reported significant improvement for the patients on indicators of stress tolerance, affect modulation, introspective abilities, quality of interpersonal relationships, and egocentricity. Improvement could be shown after short-term treatment but continued during longer-term therapy. Furthermore, researchers at the Network for Addiction Treatment Services Novadic (2003), investigating the changes in the self-perceptions of interpersonal behavior in patients with substance abuse disorder reported that significant changes on the control dimension of the ICL-R were accounted for by changes on the dimensions competitive-exploitive, aggressive-blunt, distrustful-skeptical, docile-dependent, indicating that the ICL-R is sensitive enough to evaluate change.

The present study requires replication, preferably in a sample including patients from different institutions, before more definitive conclusions can be drawn. Future researchers may wish to consider comparing specialized dynamic risk treatment programs with the 'treatment as usual' program in their particular hospital. Future research should also seek to refine measures' sensitivity to change, as the majority of the measures used to assess change in dynamic risk factors during inpatient treatment demonstrated no change.

The objective of inpatient forensic treatment is to effect changes in long-term patterns of maladaptive behavior in order to reduce violence risk. The overall trend over the course of therapy indicated that the sample as a whole did not improve on the dynamic risk factors. It is true that at baseline assessment, psychopathic patients had significantly higher ratings on a few indicators of dynamic risk factors, compared with nonpsychopathic patients. However, a PCL-R diagnosis of psychopathy was unrelated to treatment outcome. The results imply that a lack of progress should not be too easily attributed to psychopathy, and psychopathic patients should not be excluded from forensic inpatient treatment in advance. Since the treatment program was generally unsuccessful in addressing dynamic risk factors with either group of patients, no conclusions can be drawn about relative success, and this study thus has little to say either way about differential treatment-related change in persons with psychopathy. What it can say is that other patients, too, may show no change over the course of a certain type of treatment — but a different program might show differential results, so the jury is still out.

Chapter 7

PSYCHOPATHY AND SEXUAL DEVIANCE

IN TREATED RAPISTS:

ASSOCIATION WITH SEXUAL AND

NON-SEXUAL RECIDIVISM[1]

---

[1] A different version of this chapter is published as:
Hildebrand, M., Ruiter, C. de, & Vogel, V. de (2004). Psychopathy and sexual deviance in treated rapists: Association with sexual and non-sexual recidivism. *Sexual Abuse: A Journal of Research and Treatment, 16,* 1-24.
Thanks are due to Daan van Beek and Gwen Mead for assisting in data collection. We are grateful to Dennis Doren, Karl Hanson and two anonymous reviewers who commented on a previous version of this chapter.

## SUMMARY

This study investigated the role of the Psychopathy Checklist-Revised (PCL-R; Hare, 1991) and sexual deviance scores in predicting recidivism in a sample of 94 convicted rapists involuntarily admitted to a Dutch forensic psychiatric hospital between 1975 and 1996. The predictive utility of grouping offenders based on the combination of psychopathy and sexual deviance was also investigated. Furthermore, we explored the relationship between PCL-R scores and serious institutional misbehavior (i.e., unauthorized absence, physical violence, alcohol/drug use) and episodes of seclusion in response to incidents. Measures were coded from pre-release institutional records. Recidivism (reconviction) data were retrieved from the Judicial Documentation Register of the Ministry of Justice and were related to PCL-R and sexual deviance scores. The follow-up period after release ranged up to 23.5 years ($M = 11.8$ years). Base rates for sexual, violent nonsexual, violent (including sexual) and general recidivism were 34%, 47%, 55%, and 73%, respectively. Receiver Operating Characteristic (ROC) analyses provided moderate to strong support for the predictive validity of the PCL-R for inpatient disruptive behavior and recidivism outcomes. For all types of offending, offenders scoring high on the PCL-R ($\geq 26$) were significantly more often reconvicted than other offenders. The sexual deviance score was found to be a significant predictor of sexual reconviction. Survival analyses provided considerable evidence that psychopathic sex offenders with sexual deviant preferences are at substantially greater risk of committing new sexual offenses than psychopathic offenders without deviant preferences, or nonpsychopathic offenders with or without sexual deviance. The findings are discussed in terms of their practical and clinical implications.

## INTRODUCTION

Sexual assault toward adult women is a multidimensionally determined phenomenon. It encompasses a wide spectrum of behaviors targeting different types of victims in a variety of situations. Those involved in managing sex offenders, however, recognize that sex offenders are heterogeneous in their personality profiles, criminal diversity, and risk. The identification of risk factors that may be associated with recidivism in sex offenders play an important role in determining intervention strategies that best protect the community and reduce the likelihood of further victimization. To date, studies regarding the effect of interventions with these offenders have provided mixed findings (e.g., Hanson et al., 2002; Looman, Abracen, & Nicholaichuk, 2000; Marques, 1999). Sex offender treatment programs and the results of treatment outcome studies may vary not only due to their therapeutic approach, but also, for example, by the location of the treatment (e.g., prison, forensic psychiatric hospital, community), the degree of self-selection (e.g., voluntary participation or mandatory placement in a program), and the seriousness of the offender's (sex) offense history. Overall, only a small proportion of sex offenders are expected to benefit significantly from treatment (e.g., Furby, Weinrott, & Blackshaw, 1989; Hall, 1995).

In general, the recidivism rate of sex offenders is high (e.g., Doren, 1998). Overall, the observed rates for *sexual* recidivism are approximately 20% after a follow-up period of 10 years (Hanson, Morton, & Harris, in press). Recidivism rates, however, vary widely, depending on factors such as the definition and type of recidivism, whether or not offenders have completed treatment programs, the length of follow-up period after release from detention or inpatient forensic hospitalization, and type or subtype of sex offender. To illustrate, Prentky, Lee, Knight, and Cerce (1997) documented a 52% failure rate for *sexual* reoffending within their sample of extrafamilial child molesters ($N = 115$) over a 25-year at-risk period, using the definition of "charge of new sex offense". For rapists ($N = 136$), the sexual recidivism rate, as measured by a new sexual charge, was 39% over 25 years, and the corresponding reconviction rate for rapists was 24%. In addition, rapists generally show higher rates of (nonsexual) violent and general reoffending than other sex offenders (e.g., Hanson & Bussière, 1998; Marx, Miranda, & Meyerson, 1999; Prentky et al., 1997; Quinsey, Rice, & Harris, 1995).

Obviously, future behavior can never be predicted with 100% accuracy. Efforts directed at identifying factors that are predictive of future (sexual) offending, however, continue to be the focus of considerable research. In a meta-analytic review of the research, involving 61 different sex offender databases, some of which involved rapists, Hanson and Bussière (1996, 1998) found that there were different predictors for different types of recidivism. In general, the strongest predictors of *sexual* recidivism were factors related to sexual deviance and general criminal history. The single largest predictor of sexual reoffending was phallometric evidence of sexual interest in children ($r = .32$). Other predictors included clinical assessment of deviant sexual preferences ($r = .22$), prior sexual offenses ($r = .19$), and factors related to general criminality, such as antisocial personality or psychopathy ($r = .14$). Predictors of *violent nonsexual* recidivism in sex offenders were the same as those that are associated with violent recidivism in non sex offenders (e.g., age, $r = -.24$; prior violent offenses, $r = .21$; psychopathy, $r = .19$) (Andrews & Bonta, 1994; Gendreau, Little, & Goggin, 1996). However, as has been noted previously, one should be cautious in the interpretation of the data as the meta-analysis included many different types of sex offenders, such as child molesters and exhibitionists, in different settings (e.g., outpatient, inpatient, prison).

Although originally developed to function as a research diagnostic tool to identify psychopathy, considerable empirical evidence now indicates that the Hare Psychopathy Checklist-Revised (PCL-R; Hare, 1991) is an important predictor of violent and general recidivism (e.g., Hare, Clark, Grann, & Thornton, 2000; Hemphill, Hare, & Wong, 1998; Salekin, Rogers, & Sewell, 1996). Psychopathy (PCL-R) is also identified as a risk factor for sexual recidivism (Hanson & Bussière, 1996; Seto & Lalumière, 2000), although the relation between psychopathy and sexual violence is complex (Porter et al., 2000). To illustrate, in a recent evaluation of its predictive validity among sex offenders, Barbaree, Seto, Langton, and Peacock (2001) reported that PCL-R scores failed to correlate with sexual recidivism, although PCL-R total scores and Factor 2 scores showed significant correlations with any and violent (including sexual) recidivism. Similarly, AUC values for the PCL-R total score reflected moderate predictive validity for any and violent recidivism but was no better than chance for sexual recidivism specifically.

Theoretically, one might expect that certain characteristics of the (PCL-R) psychopath (e.g., sexual promiscuity, lack of concern for the welfare of others, impulsivity) would lead to higher levels of sexual activity and to nonconsenting sexual encounters. In nonpsychopathic individuals, on the other hand, concern for the victim, and lack of general propensities to use other people for one's own ends would likely to inhibit the acting out of deviant sexual preferences/fantasies. A sexually deviant psychopathic individual is less likely to show such restraint. Indeed, it is suggested that psychopathy in combination with deviant sexual arousal would be a strong predictor of sexual aggressive behavior (Hall & Hirschman, 1991; Quinsey, Lalumière, Rice, & Harris, 1995).

Recently, a number of studies have explored the relation between PCL-R psychopathy and sexual deviance, assessed with phallometric indices of deviant sexual arousal, in relation to recidivism in adult (Rice & Harris, 1997b; Serin, Mailloux, & Malcolm, 2001) and adolescent sex offenders (Gretton, McBride, Hare, O'Shaughnessy, & Kumka, 2001). Serin, Mailloux et al. (2001) reported that the combination of a high PCL-R score and deviant sexual arousal predicted *general* recidivism in a sample of rapists. Unfortunately, they did not report outcomes for sexual reoffenses. Rice and Harris (1997) reported an interaction effect of PCL-R psychopathy and sexual deviance in the prediction of *sexual* recidivism among rapists and child molesters followed for an average period of 10 years. Sexually deviant men scoring high on the PCL-R (more than 25) had a much lower survival rate (26%) than men who scored high on the PCL-R, but not on sexual deviance and those that were low on both factors. Gretton et al. (2001) found that a combination of high scores on the Hare Psychopathy Checklist: Youth Version (PCL:YV; Forth, Kosson, & Hare, in press) and phallometric evidence of deviant sexual arousal was more strongly predictive of general and violent reoffending than of sexual recidivism among adolescent sex offenders. All in all, these findings suggest that the combination of deviant sexual preferences and psychopathy puts sex offenders at particularly high risk for committing further offenses. Although past findings have been supportive of this hypothesis, further research in other, non North American samples, is needed to study the predictive validity of the relationship between psychopathy and sexual deviance with regard to criminal recidivism, with a particular emphasis on sexual reoffending.

## THE PRESENT STUDY

The main purpose of the present study was to evaluate the validity of PCL-R psychopathy for the prediction of recidivism outcomes among convicted rapists who had returned to society after (intensive) forensic psychiatric inpatient treatment. The predictive value of Factor 1 and Factor 2 of the PCL-R was also examined. The second goal of the study was to examine the relationship between PCL-R psychopathy and sexual deviance, and the degree of predictive utility when defining groups according to combinations of psychopathy (high/low) and sexual deviance (present/absent).

Contrary to the important role assigned to phallometry in the assessment of sexual deviance in North American countries, phallometry is rarely used in the Netherlands. We believe this reflects the significant differences between North American and Dutch policy regarding assessment and treatment of sex offenders. Phallometry does not fit with the historically predominantly psychodynamic orientation of Dutch forensic psychiatry. Since phallometric assessments of sexual deviance were not available for the subjects in the present study, the "Sexual Deviance" item of the Sexual Violence Risk-20 (SVR-20; Boer, Hart, Kropp, & Webster, 1997) was used for scoring sexual deviance. The SVR-20 is a 20-item structured clinical guideline for the assessment of risk for sexual violence in adult sex offenders. On the basis of previous research, we hypothesized that:

(1)     Offenders identified as psychopathic would be more likely than nonpsychopathic offenders to commit further offenses (sexual, violent nonsexual, general) after release;

(2)     With regard to sexual recidivism, psychopathic offenders with deviant sexual preferences were expected to recidivate more often and faster than other groups of offenders.

Although not the primary focus of the present study, we also explored the relationship between the PCL-R and serious institutional misbehavior. Several studies reported a generally positive (although in some studies negligible) association between PCL-R scores and disruptive behavior (see Chapter 5). However, relatively limited research has addressed this issue specifically in sex offenders, who may present unique challenges in terms of institutional management and treatment (Seto & Barbaree, 1999; Seto & Lalumière, 2000).

# METHOD

## PARTICIPANTS

Subjects ($N$ = 94) were male forensic psychiatric patients involuntarily admitted to the Dr. Henri van der Hoeven Kliniek, a Dutch forensic psychiatric hospital, between July 1975 and February 1996. Patients were convicted for rape ($n$ = 75) or sexual assault ($n$ = 19). According to the Dutch Code of Criminal Law, a criminal offender can be sentenced to a *maatregel van terbeschikkingstelling* (TBS-order) when (1) the offense committed can result in a sentence of four or more years imprisonment, with an estimated high risk of recidivism, and (2) the offender was judged to carry diminished responsibility for the offense committed due to a serious mental and/or personality disorder. The TBS-system evolved from a humanistic reform movement in criminal law, which emphasized the need for rehabilitation of mentally disordered offenders through intensive psychotherapeutic effort. The main purpose of the TBS-order is to protect society from unacceptably high risks of recidivism, directly through involuntary admission to a secure forensic psychiatric hospital, and indirectly by offering treatment to the mentally disordered offender. Treatment is aimed at structural and lasting behavior change, to allow a safe return to society. Every one or two years the court reviews the risk of reoffending to determine whether the TBS-order needs to be prolonged.

## SAMPLE CHARACTERISTICS

At admission, the mean age of the sample was 24.5 years ($SD$ = 5.5; range = 18-44). Most of the patients were White (95%). The academic and vocational background of the sample was clearly below average. Ten patients (11%) did not complete elementary school and 52 patients (55%) had no further education after elementary school. At the time of the index offense, most patients were single (79%) and without a job (56%). Eighty-two patients (89%, missing data for two patients) had been convicted at least once before (mean number of previous convictions for any crime was 4.47, $SD$ = 5.47; range = 0 - 28). The mean duration of forensic inpatient treatment was 53 months ($SD$ = 27 months; range = 2 - 156 months).

## PROCEDURE

The study had a retrospective follow-up design. With the exception of recidivism data, the study variables were coded retrospectively from institutional files. In general, the files were extensive and contained psychiatric and psychological evaluations, police records, criminal history, treatment plans and treatment evaluations, the hospital's (bi-)annual advice to the court about the need for prolongation of the TBS-order, and family background data. The files were reviewed and coded by the authors, without knowledge of recidivism data.

## ASSESSMENTS

*Psychopathy.* Psychopathy was measured using the Psychopathy Checklist-Revised (PCL-R; Hare, 1991; Dutch translation: Vertommen, Verheul, de Ruiter, & Hildebrand, 2002), a reliable and well validated (e.g., Hemphill, Hare, & Wong, 1998) 20-item structured clinical assessment instrument based on the description by Cleckley (1941/1982) of a personality style which he named psychopathy. Subjects were assigned ratings of '0' (*absent*), '1' (*some indication*), or '2' (*present*) on each of the PCL-R items, measuring characteristics as glibness/superficial charm, lack of empathy, need for stimulation/proneness to boredom, poor behavioral controls, impulsivity, and juvenile delinquency. Factor analyses have consistently found two correlated but distinct factors for the PCL-R (Hare, 1991), although there is recent evidence to suggest that a three factor solution (Cooke & Michie, 2001) better reflects the multifaceted concept of psychopathy. The two-factor model is comprised of a first factor that has been described as callous and remorseless disregard for the rights and feelings of others (Hare, 1991), consisting of eight items that measure the affective and interpersonal features of the disorder. Factor 2 consists of nine items describing a chronically unstable, impulsive, and antisocial lifestyle. Total scores can range from 0 to 40, and the recommended cut-off score for a diagnosis of psychopathy is 30 (Hare, 1991, 1996), although in European studies a cut-off score of 26 is often used to differentiate between PCL-R psychopaths and nonpsychopaths (e.g., Grann, Långström, Tengström, & Stålenheim, 1998; Rasmussen, Storsæter, & Levander, 1999; Sjöstedt & Långström, 2002). The PCL-R is completed on the basis of a semi-structured interview and file information, or on the basis of file information alone, provided that the file material is extensive and detailed. In a previous study (Hildebrand, de Ruiter, de Vogel, & van der Wolf, 2002), high interrater reliability was demonstrated for the Dutch language version of the PCL-R.

In this study, PCL-R ratings for the 94 offenders were made by a single rater (CdR or VdV) on the basis of file information only. Although the PCL-R was not designed to be used without a clinical interview, several studies (e.g., Grann et al., 1998; Wong, 1988) have shown that PCL-R scores derived from (extensive) file data can be reliable and are acceptable for research purposes. In order to establish interrater reliability of file-only PCL-R ratings, the first author independently rated a random sample of 59 files. All three raters had been extensively trained in the PCL-R, by Drs. Robert D. Hare and David Cooke in a three-day PCL-R workshop held at the Dr. Henri van der Hoeven Kliniek (October 1997) and by Drs. Robert D. Hare and Stephen D. Hart in a three-day PCL-R workshop (Nijmegen, April 2000). The interrater reliability (two independent raters) for PCL-R total and factor scores appeared to be excellent. The single measure intraclass correlation coefficient (ICC; Shrout & Fleiss, 1979; McGraw & Wong, 1996) for the PCL-R adjusted total score was .90 (ICC Factor 1 = .79, ICC Factor 2 = .80). Comparison of PCL-R categorical diagnoses among two raters showed good agreement (Cohens's κ = .66) on the absence or presence of PCL-R psychopathy (adjusted sum total score ≥ 26); in 49 of the 59 cases (83%) the raters agreed on the presence or absence of the diagnosis of psychopathy. Internal consistency for the sample ($N = 94$) was acceptable for PCL-R total (Cronbach's α = .74) and factor scores (α for Factor 1 = .78; α for Factor 2 = .80).

*Sexual deviance scores.* According to the fourth edition of the *Diagnostic and Statistical Manual of Mental Disorders* (American Psychiatric Association, 1994), sexual deviance — or deviant sexual preferences — are sexual preferences considered deviant because they are both statistically unusual and, when acted upon, likely to inflict unwarranted harm on oneself or others, such as exhibitionism, and sexual sadism. For the purpose of this study, we operationalized the presence of sexual deviance as having a score of '1' (*possibly or partially present*) or '2' (*definitely present*) on the "Sexual Deviance" item (Item 1) of the Sexual Violence Risk-20 (SVR-20; Boer et al., 1997; authorized Dutch language version: Hildebrand, de Ruiter, & van Beek, 2001), a set of professional guidelines designed to assist clinical risk assessment in sexual offenders. The scoring criteria followed the guidelines presented by the SVR-20.

The determination of sexual deviance was based on the person's documented history of offending ("pre-treatment" information, including police files and psychological and/or psychiatric assessments) and/or the patient's acknowledgement of the sexual deviance during treatment (information gathered during treatment disclosures). Any diagnosed paraphilia constituted sexual deviance in the present study, ranging from exhibitionism to sadism to pedophilia to more atypical paraphilias. Ratings had been performed earlier, as part of a study of the psychometric properties of the SVR-20 by de Vogel, de Ruiter, van Beek, and Mead (2004). In order to establish interrater reliability of the sexual deviance ratings, a random sample of 24 files coded by the third author was also coded by a second rater (a senior psychotherapist ($n$ = 9) or the second author ($n$ = 15). Comparison of sexual deviance scores among the two independent raters showed fair to good agreement (Cohens's κ = .59); in 19 of the 24 cases (79%) the raters agreed on the presence or absence of sexual deviance.

*Institutional misbehavior.* Hospital case files were reviewed by MH in order to assess three types of serious institutional misbehavior: *Unauthorized absence*, *Physical violence*, *Alcohol/drug use*. Also, episodes of seclusion in response to incidents were reviewed. All criterion measures were coded dichotomously.

*Recidivism data.* Data on recidivism were retrieved from the so-called Judicial Documentation Register of the Dutch Ministry of Justice. Recidivism was coded into four categories: (1) *Sexual* recidivism referred to whether or not the patient was reconvicted for a sexual offense, in accordance with Dutch criminal law, during the follow-up period; (2) *Violent nonsexual* recidivism referred to whether or not the patient was reconvicted for a violent nonsexual offense (e.g., attempted or completed homicide, assault, robbery); (3) *Violent* recidivism included reconvictions for both violent nonsexual and sexual offenses; (4) *General* recidivism was defined as any reconviction (including property and drug offenses) noted in the Judicial Documentation Register. Reoffending *during* the TBS-order, i.e., while the patient was still in treatment, was included as a reconviction.

All subjects were retrospectively followed from date of release from the Dr. Henri van der Hoeven Kliniek, or transfer to another hospital, to first occurrence of sexual, violent nonsexual, violent and general reoffending, or to end of follow-up (December 1, 2001). Mean follow-up time was 11.8 years (*SD* = 6 years), varying from 1.8 to 23.5 years.

## STATISTICAL ANALYSES

The predictive accuracy of the PCL-R was examined with Areas Under the Curve (AUC) in Receiver Operating Characteristics (ROC) analyses (e.g., Rice & Harris, 1995a). ROC analysis is less reliant than other statistical analyses (percentage agreement, correlation coefficient) on base rates of recidivism and the particular cut off score chosen to classify cases (Mossman, 1994; Rice & Harris, 1995a). Also, normality need not be assumed (Rice & Harris, 1995a). ROCs take the form of a plot, with the sensitivity (true positive rate) of the predictor plotted as a function of the false positive rate. The AUC of the ROC graph can be considered as an index for the overall accuracy of the predictor. Areas can range from 0 (perfect negative prediction) to .50 (chance prediction) to 1.0 (perfect positive accuracy in prediction). The AUC represents the probability that a randomly selected true recidivist would be more likely to have a high score on the instrument than a randomly selected truly non-recidivist (Mossman, 1994). An AUC of 71% indicates that there is a 71% chance that a violent individual would have a higher score on the risk measure than a nonviolent individual. Based on a comparison with the literature, AUCs in the range of .70 to .80 are considered to demonstrate moderate to large effect sizes (e.g., Rice, 1997).

The association between PCL-R psychopathy and the dichotomous (failure vs. no failure) outcome variables (i.e., types of reconviction) was examined in several ways. Chi-square was computed for the group differences in outcome (with $df = 1$, $N = 94$). We tested each chi-square with Yates' correction for continuity. A diagnosis of psychopathy was defined as a score of 26 or more on the PCL-R. Next, we computed odds ratios (OR) with 95% confidence intervals (CI) to compare the PCL-R groups on the risk for each type of recidivism. The OR indicates the degree to which the odds of committing an offense are greater for one group (i.e., psychopathic sex offenders) than for another (nonpsychopathic sex offenders). ORs greater than 3 will be considered evidence of a strong association (Douglas & Webster, 1999; Fleiss, Williams, & Dubro, 1986). In addition, we calculated ORs to examine the association between sexual deviance and recidivism.

Survival analyses were conducted to determine the likelihood of occurrence of reoffending and the average time prior to that event. Survival analysis calculates the probability of recidivating for each time period given that the offender has not yet reoffended. Once an offender recidivates, he is removed from the analysis of subsequent time periods. Survival analysis has the advantage of being able to estimate year-by-year recidivism rates even when the follow-up periods vary across offenders. The Kaplan-Meier method was used to obtain the survival curves, and the log rank statistic was used to test differences between the survival curves of the subgroups.

We also studied a number of other potential risk factors in relation to recidivism to compare the PCL-R with these other predictors of reoffending. The question was whether these variables added incrementally to the accuracy of psychopathy (PCL-R $\geq$ 26; dichotomous) in predicting recidivism outcomes. The selection of these covariates took place on an empirical (suggested by previous research, e.g., Hanson & Bussière, 1996, 1998; Salekin et al., 1996) and practical (availability) basis. The following variables were included: Age at first offense (continuous), marital status (never married; dichotomous), substance abuse/dependence (dichotomous; not included for sexual recidivism), and number of prior convictions for sexual, violent nonsexual, violent or general offenses (continuous). Cox regression analyses (Cox, 1972) were used to investigate the relationship between the independent variables and recidivism outcomes over time. To evaluate effects of predictors on survival, the Cox proportional hazards model, which assumes that the hazard ratio is invariant across time (i.e., that the effect of a predictor variable is stable over time), was used. Violation of the assumption requires the time interaction effect and ensures that the estimation of the effect of the predictor is reliable (e.g., Tabachnick & Fidell, 2001).

# RESULTS

## DESCRIPTIVE CHARACTERISTICS

The mean adjusted total score of the PCL-R for this sample was 22.2 ($SD$ = 7.3; range 8 to 36), with a median score of 22.1 and a mode of 16.0. The kurtosis of the PCL-R score was –1.028 ($SE$ = .493). PCL-R scores were normally distributed (Kolmogorov-Smirnov $Z$ = .791, $p$ = .558). The mean Factor 1 score was 7.7 ($SD$ = 3.5) and the mean Factor 2 score was 11.8 ($SD$ = 4.7). Using a cut-off score of 26 to divide patients into a psychopathic and a nonpsychopathic group, 33 patients (35.1%) fulfilled the criterion for psychopathy. When the recommended cut-off point of 30 was used (Hare, 1991), 20 patients (21.3%) were classified as 'psychopaths'.

The distribution of SVR-20 item 1 (sexual deviance) scores was as follows: 54 patients were rated '0' (*absent*), 27 were rated '1' (*possibly or partially present*), and 13 were rated '2' (*present*). Thus, 40 patients (43%) in the sample met our criterion for sexual deviance.

## BIVARIATE RELATIONSHIPS BETWEEN PCL-R SCORES AND DISRUPTIVE BEHAVIOR

Table 1 presents point-biserial correlations between PCL-R scores and the categories of disruptive behavior, and episodes of seclusion in response to incidents.

## TABLE 1

*Pearson Point-Biserial Correlations Between PCL-R Scores and Indicators of Institutional Misbehavior*

| Type of Behavior | PCL-R total | Factor 1 | Factor 2 |
|---|---|---|---|
| Unauthorized absence | .47*** | .21* | .54*** |
| Physical violence | .28** | .10 | .37*** |
| Alcohol/drugs use | .20* | .10 | .20* |
| Episodes of seclusion | .36*** | .24** | .37*** |

*Note.* PCL-R = Psychopathy Checklist-Revised. Significant correlations are in bold.
*$p$ < .05. **$p$ < .01. ***$p$ < .001.

With regard to unauthorized absence, significant correlations were found for the PCL-R total ($r_{pb}$ = .47, $p$ < .001), Factor 1 ($r_{pb}$ = .21, $p$ < .05) and Factor 2 ($r_{pb}$ = .54, $p$ < .001) scores. Physical violence was significantly related to the PCL-R total ($r_{pb}$ = .28, $p$ < .01) and Factor 2 ($r_{pb}$ = .37, $p$ < .001) score. The use of alcohol and/or drugs was also significantly related to the PCL-R total ($r_{pb}$ = .20, $p$ < .05) and Factor 2 score ($r_{pb}$ = .20, $p$ < .05). Frequency of seclusion correlated significantly with the PCL-R total ($r_{pb}$ = .36, $p$ < .001), Factor 1 ($r_{pb}$ = .24, $p$ < .01), and Factor 2 ($r_{pb}$ = .37, $p$ < .001) score. Factor 2 correlated stronger with disruptive behavior than Factor 1.

### PREDICTIVE ACCURACY OF THE PCL-R

*Institutional misbehavior.* We also conducted ROC analysis to examine the potential utility of the PCL-R to differentiate between those who were versus those who were not involved in institutional misbehavior. The AUCs demonstrating the strength of the relationship of the PCL-R with institutional misbehavior in our sample are modest to large (AUCs varying from .61 to .82), except for the association between physical violence and Factor 1 (AUC = .56) and alcohol/drug use and Factor 1 (AUC = .56). Unauthorized absence was strongly predicted by the PCL-R total (AUC = .79) and Factor 2 (AUC = .82). Both the PCL-R total (AUC = . 66) and Factor 2 (AUC = .72) score also significantly predicted physical violence, whereas the PCL-R total, Factor 1 and Factor 2 scores demonstrated a statistically significant ability to discriminate between individuals with and without episodes of seclusion. Alcohol/drug use was not significantly predicted by the PCL-R scores. Table 2 summarizes the results of these analyses for the criterion measures of interest.

**TABLE 2**

*Summary of ROC analyses for PCL-R Predictions of Institutional Misbehavior and Episodes of Seclusion in Response to Incidents*

| | AUC | SE | 95% CI |
|---|---|---|---|
| **Unauthorized absence** | | | |
| PCL-R total | .79*** | .05 | .69 - .88 |
| Factor 1 | .64* | .06 | .53 - .76 |
| Factor 2 | .82*** | .04 | .74 - .91 |
| **Physical violence** | | | |
| PCL-R total | .66** | .06 | .55 - .77 |
| Factor 1 | .56 | .06 | .45 - .68 |
| Factor 2 | .72*** | .05 | .62 - .82 |
| **Alcohol/drug use** | | | |
| PCL-R total | .61 | .06 | .49 - .72 |
| Factor 1 | .56 | .06 | .45 - .68 |
| Factor 2 | .60 | .06 | .49 - .72 |
| **Seclusion** | | | |
| PCL-R total | .71*** | .05 | .61 - .82 |
| Factor 1 | .64* | .06 | .53 - .75 |
| Factor 2 | .73*** | .05 | .63 - .83 |

*Note.* AUC = Area under the curve. SE = Standard error. CI = Confidence interval.
*p < .05. **p < .01. ***p < .001.

*Recidivism.* The AUCs demonstrating the strength of the relationship of the PCL-R with recidivism in our sample are modest to moderate (AUCs varying from .62 to .74), except for the association between violent nonsexual reconviction and Factor 1 (AUC = .55). Both the PCL-R total and Factor 1 score significantly, albeit moderately, predicted *sexual* reconviction with an AUC of the ROC of .65. *Violent nonsexual* and *violent* reconviction was significantly predicted by the PCL-R total and Factor 2 scores. PCL-R total, Factor 1 and Factor 2 scores demonstrated a statistically significant ability to discriminate between individuals with and without *general* reconviction during the time-at-risk period. Table 3 summarizes the results of the ROC analyses for the four types of recidivism.

TABLE 3
*Recidivism Predicted by the Psychopathy Checklist-Revised (N = 94)*

|  | AUC | SE | 95% CI | *r* |
|---|---|---|---|---|
| **Sexual** | | | | |
| PCL-R total | .68** | .06 | .56 - .80 | .24* |
| Factor 1 | .67** | .06 | .56 - .78 | .23* |
| Factor 2 | .65* | .06 | .53 - .77 | .18 |
| **Violent nonsexual** | | | | |
| PCL-R total | .66** | .06 | .55 - .77 | .28** |
| Factor 1 | .55 | .06 | .44 - .67 | .09 |
| Factor 2 | .68** | .06 | .58 - .79 | .33** |
| **Violent (including sexual)** | | | | |
| PCL-R total | .70** | .05 | .59 - .80 | .32** |
| Factor 1 | .62 | .06 | .51 - .73 | .19 |
| Factor 2 | .69** | .06 | .58 - .83 | .31** |
| **General** | | | | |
| PCL-R total | .74** | .05 | .63 - .84 | .30** |
| Factor 1 | .67** | .06 | .55 - .80 | .22* |
| Factor 2 | .71** | .06 | .58 - .83 | .27** |

*Note.* AUC = Area under the curve. SE = Standard error. CI = Confidence interval. Pearson point-biserial correlations between PCL-R scores and the dichotomous outcome variables are also presented, as they are easily understood, and to facilitate comparison with the results of other studies.
*p < .05. **p < .01.

## PSYCHOPATHY AND RECIDIVISM RATES

*Chi-square.* By the end of the follow-up period, which ranged up to 23,5 years, 32 of the 94 sex offenders (34%) had been reconvicted for a *sexual* offense. A total of 44 (47%) subjects were reconvicted for a *violent nonsexual* offense; 53 (55%) for a *violent* offense, and 69 (73%) for a *general* offense.

Failure rates for psychopathic and nonpsychopathic sex offenders are depicted in Table 4. For psychopathic offenders, the failure rate for sexual recidivism was 55%, for violent nonsexual recidivism 64%, for violent recidivism 76%, and for general recidivism 91%. For nonpsychopathic sex offenders, failure rates were 23%, 38%, 44%, and 64%, respectively. It is clear that psychopathic offenders were more likely to recidivate than nonpsychopathic offenders. The group differences using Yates' correction for continuity ($df$ = 1, $N$ = 94 in each comparison) were significant for sexual failure, $\chi^2$ = 8.17, $p$ < .05; violent nonsexual failure, $\chi^2$ = 4.79, $p$ < .05; violent, $\chi^2$ = 7.37, $p$ < .05, and general failure, $\chi^2$ = 6.66, $p$ < .05.

*Odds ratios.* The odds of reconviction given patient's PCL-R scores above or equal to/ below 26 on the PCL-R were as follows ($df$ = 1, $N$ = 94 in each comparison; 95% confidence intervals in brackets) for each type of recidivism: sexual recidivism, 4.03 (1.62-9.99), $\chi^2$ = 9.52, $p$ < .01; violent nonsexual recidivism, 2.89 (1.20-6.96), $\chi^2$ = 5.78, $p$ < .05; violent recidivism, 3.94 (1.53-10.10), $\chi^2$ = 8.59, $p$ < .01; general recidivism, 5.64 (1.53-20.63), $\chi^2$ = 7.98, $p$ < .01. That is, offenders with PCL-R scores $\geq$ 26 were more likely to be convicted for all types of offenses.

TABLE 4

*Base Rates (In Percentages), With Survival Probability Rates in Brackets, of Four Types of Reconviction For Sex Offenders, Subdivided by Psychopathy and Sexual Deviance*

| | | | Type of recidivism | | | | | | |
|---|---|---|---|---|---|---|---|---|---|
| | *N* | Sexual | | Violent Nonsexual | | Violent | | General | |
| **Total sample** | 94 | 34 | (45) | 47 | (58) | 55 | (68) | 73 | (100) |
| **PCL-R score** | | | | | | | | | |
| PCL-R ≥ 26 | 33 | 55 | (60) | 64 | (69) | 76 | (78) | 91 | (100) |
| PCL-R < 26 | 61 | 23 | (35) | 38 | (50) | 44 | (61) | 64 | (100) |
| **Sexual deviance** | | | | | | | | | |
| Deviant | 40 | 48 | (56) | 47 | (55) | 62 | (69) | 72 | (87) |
| Nondeviant | 54 | 20 | (28) | 46 | (60) | 48 | (62) | 70 | (84) |
| **Psychopathy and sexual deviance** | | | | | | | | | |
| High PCL-R / deviant | 17 | 82 | (85) | 59 | (69) | 82 | (82) | 94 | (100) |
| High PCL-R / nondeviant | 16 | 25 | (25) | 69 | (72) | 69 | (71) | 88 | (88) |
| Low PCL-R / deviant | 23 | 30 | (38) | 39 | (44) | 52 | (58) | 65 | (100) |
| Low PCL-R / nondeviant | 38 | 18 | (35) | 37 | (58) | 39 | (61) | 63 | (75) |

*Note.* PCL-R=Psychopathy Checklist-Revised. In survival analysis, the cumulative survival function represents the proportion of participants remaining free of an offense as a function of time since release. That is, survival is depicted as not having failed, although here we refer to its inverse, namely, failure.

*Survival analyses.* Survival analyses revealed that the survival functions of psychopathic (*M* = 10.8) and nonpsychopathic offenders (*M* = 16.8) differed significantly with respect to *sexual* recidivism (log rank = 6.15, *p* < .05). Psychopathic offenders had also significantly worse survival times than nonpsychopathic offenders for *violent* reoffending (*M* = 7.3 vs. *M* = 12 years; log rank = 5.74, *p* < .05). Also, psychopathic offenders had worse survival times than nonpsychopathic offenders for violent nonsexual (*M* = 9.7 vs. *M* = 13.6 years; log rank = 3.59, *p* = .06), and general recidivism (*M* = 5.3 vs. *M* = 8.3 years; log rank = 3.17, *p* = .07). However, these differences failed to reach statistical significance.

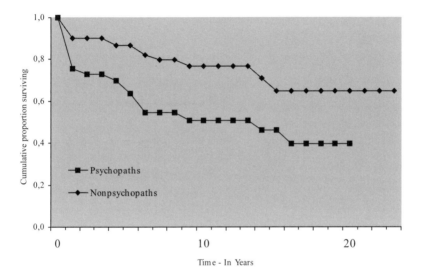

**FIGURE 1**

*Kaplan-Meier Survival Curves for Sexual Recidivism for Psychopathic (PCL-R ≥ 26) and Nonpsychopathic (PCL-R < 26) Rapists*

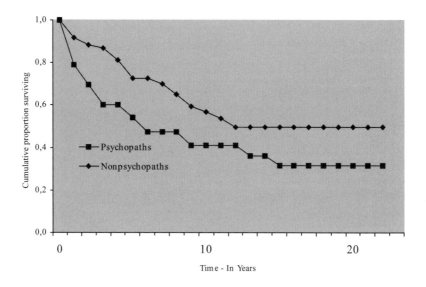

**FIGURE 2**

*Kaplan-Meier Survival Curves for Violent Nonsexual Recidivism for Psychopathic (PCL-R ≥ 26) and Nonpsychopathic (PCL-R < 26) Rapists*

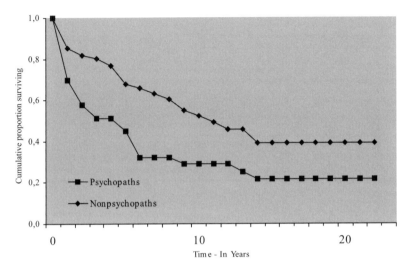

**FIGURE 3**

*Kaplan-Meier Survival Curves for Violent Recidivism for Psychopathic (PCL-R ≥ 26) and Nonpsychopathic (PCL-R < 26) Rapists*

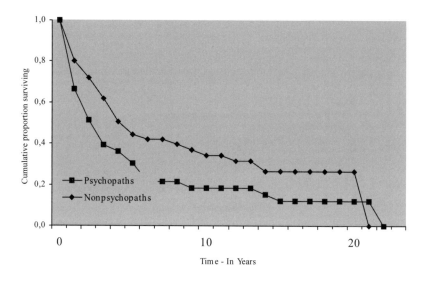

**FIGURE 4**

*Kaplan-Meier Survival Curves for General Recidivism for Psychopathic (PCL-R ≥ 26) and Nonpsychopathic (PCL-R < 26) Rapists*

*Cox regression analyses.* Results of the regression analyses to predict recidivism outcomes are presented in Table 5.

TABLE 5

*Summary of Cox Regression Analyses Using the PCL-R and Potential Risk Factors to Predict Types of Recidivism*

| | β | *SE* β | Wald | $e^B$ | 95% CI $e^B$ |
|---|---|---|---|---|---|
| **Sexual reoffending**[a] | | | | | |
| *Block 1* | | | | | |
| PCL-R | .90 | .36 | 6.38 * | 2.46 | 1.22 – 4.96 |
| *Block 2* | | | | | |
| PCL-R | .65 | .38 | 2.92 | 1.90 | .91 – 3.99 |
| Age at first offense | -.01 | .04 | .16 | .99 | .92 – 1.06 |
| Marital status | .97 | .50 | 3.78 * | 2.63 | 1.00 – 6.97 |
| Prior sexual offenses | .68 | .20 | 11.25 *** | 1.98 | 1.33 – 2.95 |
| **Violent nonsexual reoffending**[b] | | | | | |
| *Block 1* | | | | | |
| PCL-R | .77 | .31 | 6.09 ** | 2.15 | 1.17 – 3.94 |
| *Block 2* | | | | | |
| PCL-R | .45 | .34 | 1.75 | 1.57 | .80 – 3.09 |
| Age at first offense | -.04 | .04 | .89 | .96 | .88 – 1.04 |
| Marital status | .17 | .37 | .21 | 1.19 | .57 – 2.47 |
| Substance abuse/dependence | .85 | .34 | 6.13 * | 2.33 | 1.19 – 4.55 |
| Prior violent nonsexual offenses | .24 | .11 | 4.52 * | 1.27 | 1.02 – 1.59 |
| **Violent reoffending**[c] | | | | | |
| *Block 1* | | | | | |
| PCL-R | .85 | .28 | 8.85 ** | 2.33 | 1.34 – 4.07 |
| *Block 2* | | | | | |
| PCL-R | .57 | .31 | 3.45 | 1.77 | .97 – 3.23 |
| Age at first offense | -.04 | .04 | 1.20 | .96 | .89 – 1.03 |
| Marital status | .24 | .34 | .48 | 1.27 | .65 – 2.46 |
| Substance abuse/dependence | .39 | .30 | 1.66 | 1.47 | .82 – 2.64 |
| Prior violent offenses | .17 | .09 | 3.55 | 1.18 | .99 – 1.41 |

(*table continues*)

**TABLE 5** (*cont.*)

|  | β | *SE* β | Wald | $e^B$ | 95% CI $e^B$ |
|---|---|---|---|---|---|
| **General reoffending**[d] | | | | | |
| *Block 1* | | | | | |
| PCL-R | .57 | .25 | 5.38 * | 1.77 | 1.09 – 2.88 |
| *Block 2* | | | | | |
| PCL-R | .57 | .26 | 3.69 | 1.66 | .99 - 2.79 |
| Age at first offense | .00 | .04 | .00 | 1.00 | .93 – 1.08 |
| Marital status | .28 | .29 | .92 | 1.32 | .75 – 2.32 |
| Substance abuse/dependence | .05 | .27 | .03 | 1.05 | .62 – 1.76 |
| Prior offenses | .06 | .02 | 7.24 ** | 1.06 | 1.02 – 1.10 |

*Note.* Due to missing values, $N = 90$ for all regression analyses.
[a] $\chi^2 (1) = 6.82$ at Block 1, $p < .01$; $\Delta\chi^2 (3) = 14.92$ at Block 2, $p < .01$ ; for the final equation, $\chi^2 (4) = 23.74, p < .001$.
[b] $\chi^2 (1) = 6.38$ at Block 1, $p < .05$; $\Delta\chi^2 (4) = 14.52$ at Block 2, $p < .01$; for the final equation, $\chi^2 (4) = 23.16, p < .001$.
[c] $\chi^2 (1) = 9.37$ at Block 1, $p < .01$; $\Delta\chi^2 (4) = 9.08$ at Block 2, $p = .059$; for the final equation, $\chi^2 (4) = 18.82, p < .01$.
[d] $\chi^2 (1) = 5.53$ at Block 1, $p < .05$; $\Delta\chi^2 (4) = 7.54$ at Block 2, $p = .110$; for the final equation, $\chi^2 (4) = 15.28, p < .01$.
* $p \le .05$. ** $p \le 01$. *** $p \le 001$.

For all types of recidivism, the PCL-R dichotomous category variable was entered in Block 1. In Block 2, the other variables were forced into the model. For *sexual* recidivism, the PCL-R entered in the first Block accounted for a significant portion of the variance. With the entry of Age at first offense, Marital status and Prior sexual convictions in Block 2, there was a significant increment in the amount of variance explained. Marital status and Prior sexual convictions accounted for unique variance in sexual recidivism. For *violent nonsexual* reoffending, psychopathy entered in Block 1 accounted for a significant portion of the variance. The addition of the predictors Substance abuse/dependence and Prior violent nonsexual convictions produced a significant increment in the amount of variance explained. After addition of the other risk factors, the PCL-R failed to reach conventional levels of statistical significance ($p = .187$) at Block 2. *Violent* recidivism (i.e., including sexual) was significantly predicted by the PCL-R at Block 1. The addition of the predictors in Block 2 failed to produce a significant increment in the amount of variance explained by the PCL-R alone. Psychopathy ($p = .063$) and Prior violent offenses ($p =$

.059), however, remained as near-significant predictors. Finally, for *general* recidivism, the PCL-R entered in the first Block accounted for a significant portion of the variance. Of the variables added in Block 2, only Total number of prior convictions produced a significant increment in the amount of variance explained by the PCL-R alone, with Psychopathy almost reaching significance ($p = .055$).

## SEXUAL DEVIANCE SCORES AND RECIDIVISM

A total of 19 (48%) of the 40 sexually deviant offenders were convicted for at least one *sexual* reoffense, whereas 11 (20%) of the 54 offenders without deviant sexual preferences were reconvicted for a sexual offense (Table 2). For *violent nonsexual* offenses, rates were 47% and 46%; for *violent* recidivism, 62% and 48%; for *general* recidivism, 72% and 70%, respectively. As expected, odds ratios revealed that the presence of sexual deviance was significantly associated with an increased risk of reconviction for a *sexual* offense, increasing the risk with a factor of over 3 ($OR = 3.54$, 95% CI = 1.43 – 8.77; $\chi^2 = 7.83$, $p = .005$). The survival functions of sexually deviant offenders ($M = 12.8$ years) and nondeviant offenders ($M = 17.6$ years) differed significantly with regard to *sexual* recidivism (log rank = 5.57, $p < .05$). For violent nonsexual, violent, and general recidivism, no significant differences were found.

## PSYCHOPATHY AND SEXUAL DEVIANCE IN RELATION TO SEXUAL RECIDIVISM

PCL-R psychopaths and nonpsychopaths were further subdivided on the basis of presence or absence of deviant sexual preferences to create the following four groups: psychopathic/deviant ($n = 17$), psychopathic/nondeviant ($n = 16$), nonpsychopathic /deviant ($n = 23$), and nonpsychopathic/nondeviant ($n = 38$). For the psychopathic/deviant group, the failure rate for a sexual reconviction during the follow-up period was extremely high, i.e., 82%. For the psychopathic/nondeviant group, it was 25%; for the nonpsychopathic/deviant group, it was 30% and for the nonpsychopathic/nondeviant group, it was 18% (Table 2).

Although the number of subjects in each subgroup was small, a clear interaction between psychopathy and sexual deviance was found for *sexual* recidivism (see Figure 1). PCL-R psychopaths with deviant sexual preferences recidivated much faster and more often (i.e., at a higher rate) than subjects in the other three groups (log rank = 12.06, $p$ < .05). On average, psychopathic/ deviant offenders failed after 9.4 years. Psychopathic/nondeviant offenders and nonpsychopathic/deviant offenders had similar survival times ($M$ = 15.6 and 15.7 years, respectively), whereas subjects in the psychopathic/nondeviant group, on average, failed after 17.3 years. No other significant interaction effects were found.

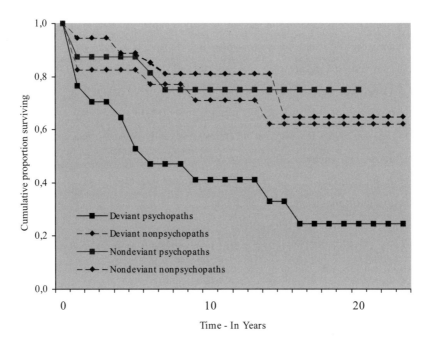

**FIGURE 5**
*Kaplan-Meier Survival Curves for Sexual Recidivism for Psychopathic (PCL-R ≥ 26) and Nonpsychopathic (PCL-R < 26) Rapists Subdivided into Those With and Without Deviant Sexual Preferences*

## ADDITIONAL ANALYSES

*Failure to complete treatment.* Only 30 patients (32%) completed the treatment provided in the hospital. For 33 patients, the court ended the TBS-order *against* the hospital's advice and 28 patients were readmitted to another forensic psychiatric institution. In most cases, the reason for readmission was that further treatment was deemed impossible due to a disturbed relationship between the patient and hospital staff.

Chi-square analyses revealed that sex offenders who did not complete the treatment provided in the hospital were more likely to recidivate with a sexual offense than offenders who had completed their hospital treatment. The group difference using Yates' correction for continuity was significant, $\chi^2$ (1, 94) = 4.84, $p$ < .05. Interestingly, 16 of the 17 psychopathic/deviant offenders had ended treatment prematurely; 14 of these 16 offenders recidivated with a sexual offense. Over the period, the survival rate between groups was significantly different. Sex offenders who had ended their hospital treatment prematurely began reoffending earlier after their release and continued to reoffend with a sexual offense throughout the entire follow-up period (log rank = 4.19, $p$ < .05). For violent nonsexual, violent, and general recidivism, no significant differences between treatment completers and noncompleters were found.

## DISCUSSION

The present study explored the relevance of PCL-R psychopathy and sexual deviance, in relation to sexual, violent nonsexual, violent and general recidivism (i.e., reconvictions) in a Dutch sample of offenders convicted for rape or sexual assault, involuntarily admitted to a forensic psychiatric hospital. Secondly, the study investigated the predictive utility of defining offenders according to combinations of psychopathy and sexual deviance. We also explored the relationship between PCL-R scores and disruptive behavior during inpatient treatment. Retrospective PCL-R ratings and sexual deviance scores were based on extensive file-based data from various sources. The interrater reliability of the file-based PCL-R ratings was high. In general, the high levels of reliability found in the present study are consistent with those documented by other researchers using file material only (e.g., Grann et al., 1998), and further support the use of file-only ratings for research objectives.

In our sample, the sexual reconviction rate was 34%, over an average follow-up period of 11.8 years. In other studies (Proulx et al., 1997; Rice, Harris, & Quinsey, 1990; Quinsey et al. 1995; Sjöstedt & Långström, 2002) the reported sexual reconviction rate was somewhat lower (± 21 - 28%). Differences in sexual reconviction rates may be due to the shorter follow-up period in these studies. With longer follow-up periods, the rate increases to 35% - 45% after 15 to 25 years (Prentky et al., 1997; Rice & Harris, 1997b). Doubtless, the reported recidivism rates are very conservative, because a substantial proportion of sex offenses remains undetected (Bonta & Hanson, 1994; Doren, 1998). Our findings further indicate that rapists did not limit their recidivism to sexual offenses. In fact, they were more likely to be convicted for a new violent nonsexual offense, which is in line with previous research (e.g., Prentky et al., 1997; Sjöstedt & Långström, 2002); 44 subjects (47%) were reconvicted for a violent nonsexual offense.

The present results provide moderate to strong support for the predictive validity of the PCL-R for inpatient misconduct and recidivism outcomes. Consistent with earlier research in other forensic and correctional samples (e.g., Edens, Buffington-Vollum, Colwell, Johnson, & Johnson, 2002; Hare & McPherson, 1984; Heilbrun et al., 1998; see also Chapter 5), these results support the validity of PCL-R psychopathy as a significant correlate of different forms of disruptive behavior specifically among rapists. Given the relatively limited research that has been conducted on the institutional adjustment of this particular subgroup of offenders, these findings are important in that they indicate that psychopathic traits are associated not only with *reconviction* among rapists but also with institutional misbehavior during forensic treatment.

Following their release from a forensic psychiatric hospital, rapists with high PCL-R scores appeared to be at particular risk for reoffending (sexual, violent nonsexual, violent, and general). Overall, the results are consistent with other studies that have examined the association of PCL-R psychopathy recidivism outcomes of sex offenders (e.g., Serin et al., 2001). It was found that both PCL-R Factor 1 and Factor 2 were related to the criterion variables: Factor 2 showed significant predictive validity for risk of sexual and violent nonsexual reoffending, whereas Factor 1 significantly predicted risk of sexual and general reoffending. Our finding that the predictive validity of Factor 2 is higher than that of Factor 1 for violent nonsexual and violent reconviction, is in line with previous research (e.g., Grann, Långström, Tengström, & Kullgren, 1999; Salekin et al., 1996), indicating that it is the characteristics associated with a chronically unstable, socially deviant lifestyle, rather than those associated with the selfish, callous, and remorseless use of others that predict nonsexual recidivism. Moreover, survival analyses showed that violent (including sexual) offenses following release occurred significantly earlier for psychopaths, compared to nonpsychopaths. Psychopathic rapists also had worse survival times than nonpsychopathic offenders for *sexual*, *violent nonsexual* and *general* reoffending. The difference approached significance for sexual and violent nonsexual recidivism. Thus, in general, our first hypothesis (i.e., offenders identified as psychopathic would be more likely than nonpsychopathic offenders to commit further offenses after release) was confirmed.

Consistent with the results of the Hanson and Bussière (1998) meta-analysis, the total number of prior convictions (sexual, violent nonsexual, general) was found to be a significant predictor of recidivism (sexual, violent nonsexual, general, respectively), accounting for a unique portion of the variance in this outcome while controlling for psychopathy. In addition, marital status was found to be a predictor of sexual recidivism, whereas substance abuse/dependence remained as the only significant predictor for violent nonsexual reoffending, after controlling for psychopathy. Contrary, age at first offense and marital status could not predict violent nonsexual, violent or general reconviction equally well or better in this sample than PCL-R psychopathy.

Dividing subjects according to presence or absence of sexual deviance revealed that the presence of deviant sexual preferences was significantly related to an increased risk of reconviction for a sexual offense. Also, the first reoffense in offenders with deviant sexual preferences occurred significantly earlier than in those without deviant sexual preferences. To the best of our knowledge, this is the first study providing initial evidence for the usefulness of item 1 of the SVR-20 to predict sexual recidivism in rapists. A structured clinical judgment approach to the assessment of deviant sexual preferences resulted in highly similar findings as obtained with the traditional phallometric approach. Sex offenders are well known for their tendency to deny and distort their true motives and actual offense behavior (e.g., Maletzky, 1996; Marshall, 1994; Ward, McCormack, Hudson, & Polaschek, 1997). Thus, phallometric assessment is generally considered desirable for the assessment of sexual deviance, because it is thought to circumvent possibly distortive processes. The present findings point at the feasibility of using the structured clinical judgment approach of the SVR-20 to assess sexual deviance, in a less intrusive manner. Although promising, the present findings should be viewed as tentative and need to be replicated in independent samples. For example, it might very well be that the validity of the SVR-20 assessment of sexual deviance is highly dependent on the quality of file information on which the assessment is based. In our case, most files were quite extensive, with criminal history data, verbatim victim statements, and treatment progress reports. Less complete file information might compromise the validity of the SVR-20 ratings.

One of our most important findings is that psychopathic rapists with deviant sexual preferences recidivated more often and faster with a sexual offense than other groups of rapists. Although psychopathy and sexual deviance were, by themselves, related to sexual recidivism, the present findings offer considerable evidence that the combination of psychopathy and sexual deviance is of special importance in the prediction of sexual violence. Fourteen of the 17 offenders (82%) in the psychopathic/sexual deviance group recidivated with a sexual offense. Despite the small sample sizes, survival analysis provided considerable evidence that psychopathic sex offenders with sexual deviant preferences are at much greater risk of committing new sexual offenses than psychopathic sex offenders without deviant preferences and nonpsychopathic sex offenders (with or without a diagnosis of sexual deviance). These results confirm Hanson and Bussiere's argument (1998) that the risk for sexual violence should be considered independently of risk for other forms of violence. Similar results supporting the value of considering the 'bad combination' of PCL-R psychopathy and sexual deviance (measured phallometrically) for the prediction of sexual violence have been reported by Rice and Harris (1997b). However, this effect has been difficult to replicate across studies. For example, Gretton et al. (2001) and Hanson & Harris (2000) did not find the interaction for sexual recidivism, while Gretton et al. (2001) found that a combination of high scores on the PCL:Youth Version and phallometric evidence of deviant sexual arousal was predictive of general and violent reoffending. Serin et al. (2001) reported that the combination of a high PCL-R score and deviant sexual arousal predicted *general* recidivism in a sample of rapists (no outcomes for sexual reoffenses were reported). In the present study, no significant interaction effects were found for violent nonsexual and general recidivism.

In general, our findings suggest that a combination of deviant sexual preferences and psychopathy puts sex offenders at particularly high risk for committing further sexual offenses. Replication of these results with a larger sample of sex offenders is important, including samples from other Dutch forensic psychiatric institutions. Furthermore, our data underscore the importance of considering both psychopathy and sexual deviance when determining treatment intensity and degree of security required for individual patients (Serin et al., 2001). Andrews and Bonta (1994; see also Andrews et al., 1990) have argued that offenders that pose the highest risk should receive the highest level of security and the most intensive form of treatment. In general, high security can be provided in inpatient forensic settings. However, appropriate treatment for the group of psychopathic/deviant sex offenders is not available at this time. On the contrary, several studies have pointed out that providing (standard) treatment to psychopathic sex offenders may be counterproductive and may even lead to increased offending. Seto & Barbaree (1999), for example, examined the relationship between psychopathy and performance in treatment in terms of recidivism outcomes in a sample of 216 sex offenders who participated in an institutional treatment program for sex offenders. The program followed a relapse prevention model and provided treatment in daily 3-hour groups sessions over a 5-month period. It was found that the group of sex offenders with PCL-R scores above 15 (median split) who were rated as having demonstrated 'good' treatment behavior (i.e., participation in group sessions, completion of homework, attainment of treatment targets, and positive scores on global clinical ratings of motivation and change) were the most likely to reoffend. According to the authors, the results suggested that "good treatment behavior should not be considered when making management decisions, especially for men who score higher on the PCL-R" (p. 1245). In an extended follow-up of the sample, which increased the average follow-up period from 2.7 to 5.2 years, however, Barbaree, Seto, & Langton (2001), found that the interaction effect between the PCL-R and treatment behavior was no longer evident, although the association between the PCL-R and serious recidivism remained significant. Looman, Abracen, Serin, and Marquis (2002) used a similar design to examine recidivism outcomes for a sample of sex offenders ($N = 102$) who had participated in an institutional program for sex offenders. Using survival analysis, Looman et al. (2002) found that those with PCL-R scores > 25 and ratings of good progress in treatment reoffended seriously (i.e., violently or sexually) at a significantly faster rate than either of the groups with lower PCL-R scores. The failure rate for the two PCL-R groups, however, did not differ. Note that none of the three studies described above examined the association between the variables (and their interaction effect) and *sexual* recidivism.

A number of authors have discussed the need for the development and scientific evaluation of special treatment programs for psychopaths (e.g., Wallace, Vitale, & Newman, 1999; Wong, 2000). However, until now, the treatment options for (PCL-R) psychopaths are limited. We believe that the current findings point at the need for Dutch policy makers in the criminal justice field to reconsider the rehabilitation doctrine of the TBS-order for some high risk rapists — we may just not have the treatment means at this time, to allow a safe return to society for a *particular category* of rapists. One possible implication of such a conclusion is that deviant psychopathic rapists will have to be excluded from treatment programs. However, this is a "questionable extrapolation of the existing data" (Serin & Brown, 2000, p. 254) and inconsistent with the principle of treatment responsiveness (Andrews & Bonta, 1994). Nevertheless, the present findings suggest that (deviant) psychopathic rapists are highly resistant to treatment and tend to exhibit disruptive and other types of negative behavior in the context of treatment. Consistent with this pessimism, there is a general lack of empirical evidence indicating a positive effect of treatment programs on psychopaths (e.g., Blackburn, 1993; Hare, 1996, Lösel, 1998). On the other hand, there is little empirical evidence to suggest psychopaths are untreatable either (e.g., Hemphill & Hart, 2002). Considering the lack of empirical support for current sex offender programs for psychopaths and the potential of iatrogenic effects of providing treatment to psychopaths, we strongly advise that treatment programs offered to psychopathic rapists be carefully evaluated using a methodologically sound research design.

Interestingly, offenders who failed to complete treatment (68%) were at higher risk for sexual recidivism than those who completed treatment. In the past, Hanson and Bussière (1998) have reported in their meta-analysis that sex offenders who failed to attend or who dropped out of treatment were at higher risk for both sexual and general recidivism than those who successfully completed treatment. Contrary to Hanson and Bussière (1998), we did not find a relationship between treatment completion and general recidivism. Reduced risk could be due to treatment effectiveness; alternately, high-risk offenders may be those most likely to quit, or be terminated from treatment (Hanson & Bussière, 1998). In our study, for example, 16 of the 17 psychopathic/deviant offenders (i.e., high-risk cases) had ended treatment prematurely, mainly because of a disturbed relationship between the patient and hospital staff; 14 of these 16 offenders recidivated with a sexual offense. The design of the present study does not permit an inference about treatment efficacy per se. Instead, it suggests that a rapist's completion versus failure to complete treatment represents potentially useful information for the purpose of appraising risk.

Regarding generalization, all subjects in the present retrospective follow-up study were convicted for rape or sexual assault and treated in a single Dutch forensic psychiatric hospital. Although our sample is representative of Dutch sex offenders with a TBS-order, it is not of sex offenders in general. Previous research (de Vogel et al., 2004) has shown that our sample mainly includes medium-high to high risk cases, as measured by means of the Static-99 (Hanson & Thornton, 1999), an actuarial sex offender risk scale.

Several (methodological) limitations deserve attention. First of all, the sample size of the study was rather small. Larger samples would have resulted in increased power. However, this is considered a relatively minor problem given that there is such a paucity of research on recidivism of sex offenders in the Netherlands. Indeed, no prior study has examined the predictive validity of the PCL-R among Dutch sex offenders. In addition, prior published studies examining rapists/sexual assaulters have been similarly restricted by relatively limited sample sizes (e.g., Sjöstedt & Långström, 2002). In fact, despite the limited power available, the current study found evidence of the hypothesized moderate to large differences between PCL-groups in the expected direction.

Furthermore, one might argue that it would have been preferable to use a prospective design, although the retrospective follow-up or postdictive design used in the current study prevented the assessments from being confounded with outcome measures of recidivism. Indeed, several studies have used archival follow-up procedures in retrospective studies and detected sufficient base rates of recidivism to detect moderate to large effect sizes (e.g., Rice et al., 1990; Sjöstedt & Långström, 2002). Furthermore, the length of the follow-up period can be considered a strength since it has been shown that studies with a follow-up period of less than five years underestimate long-term recidivism (e.g., Prentky et al., 1997).

Another limitation concerns the penal records that were requested from the Ministry of Justice. The Dutch Criminal Law (Act of Judicial Documentation, section 7) states that offenses that have been committed over 20 years ago have to be removed from the register. Although the average follow-up period in the presented study was almost 12 years, some individual cases of re-offending may have gone undetected as a result of being removed from the official records. Finally, the files that were used in this retrospective study varied in content and quality. For example, the individual course of treatment within the forensic hospital was documented more elaborately as the years proceeded. This may have influenced PCL-R and sexual deviance ratings. Also, some files included additional information such as statements of victims or a deposition of the offender.

In conclusion, this study contributes to a growing body of research suggesting that not all rapists be equally likely to reoffend. Research has established that psychopathy is related to sexual and nonsexual violent recidivism, but there is building evidence that, with regard to sexual recidivism, comprehensive assessment should consider the combination of psychopathy and sexual deviance. Further research is needed to determine whether these factors are changeable by treatment.

# CHAPTER 8

# GENERAL DISCUSSION

## SUMMARY

Chapter 8 concludes the present thesis. First, the major findings are summarized and discussed. Subsequently, we discuss treatment-relevant motivational deficits that characterize psychopathic patients, and some of their motivational strengths. Next, some limitations of the research presented in this thesis are discussed, recommendations for clinical practice are given, and suggestions for further research on psychopathy in Dutch forensic psychiatry are outlined.

## RESEARCH QUESTIONS ADDRESSED IN THIS THESIS

This study was designed to examine the role of psychopathy in forensic psychiatric patients involuntarily admitted to the Dr. Henri van der Hoeven Kliniek, a forensic psychiatric hospital in Utrecht, the Netherlands, using the Hare Psychopathy Checklist-Revised (PCL-R). The following five main research questions were addressed and studied in a sample of forensic psychiatric patients under the TBS-order in the Netherlands:

(1)     What is the reliability and factor structure of the Dutch language version of the PCL-R?

(2)     What is the association between psychopathy and DSM-IV Axis I and Axis II disorders?

(3)     What is the predictive power of psychopathy for inpatient disruptive behavior?

(4)     What is the relationship between psychopathy and change in dynamic risk factors during forensic psychiatric treatment?

(5)     Do rapists identified as psychopathic recidivate more and faster than nonpsychopathic rapists following the termination of treatment?

## MAIN RESEARCH FINDINGS

Since results of the separate studies have been reported and discussed in detail in the previous chapters, only main issues will be reviewed in this section.

### RELIABILITY AND FACTOR STRUCTURE

In Chapter 3 it is shown that the Dutch language version of the PCL-R can be reliably rated by trained professionals, based on the Dutch translation of the semi-structured interview schedule designed by Hare (1991) and a review of all the collateral information available upon admission to the hospital. We also found good to excellent reliabilities for PCL-R ratings based on *file information only* (Chapter 7). In general, the high levels of reliability found in the present study are consistent with those documented by other researchers.

PREVALENCE OF PSYCHOPATHY

Does psychopathy frequently occur in Dutch mentally disordered offenders involuntarily admitted to a forensic psychiatric hospital? We demonstrated that psychopathy is a quite common disorder: Approximately 30% of the male forensic psychiatric patients were classified as psychopathic, using a PCL-R cut-off score of 26.

DIAGNOSTIC VALIDITY

*Association with DSM-IV Axis I disorders.* A diagnosis of PCL-R psychopathy was positively associated with drug abuse/dependence and alcohol abuse/dependence. On the other hand, patients with a diagnosis of PCL-R psychopathy were more than three times less likely to receive a diagnosis of any Axis I disorder other than alcohol or other substance use disorders. Similarly, these patients were about three times less likely to receive a diagnosis of paraphilic disorder.

*Association with DSM-IV Axis II disorders.* Psychopathy was significantly positively related to Cluster B personality disorders (PDs). Most psychopathic patients had a DSM-IV antisocial PD (i.e., 88%); the reverse was not true. PCL-R scores were also positively correlated with dimensional scores of paranoid, borderline, and narcissistic PD, and with conduct disorder (below 15 years of age) and antisocial behavior since age 15. In general, these results are consistent with previous research, providing further evidence for the cross-cultural validity of the PCL-R (Chapter 4).

PREDICTIVE VALIDITY

To be clinically relevant for the treatment of TBS-patients, it is important that the PCL-R score has significant power to predict (1) the course of treatment or (2) treatment outcome. Ideally, to improve overall treatment outcome, psychopathy would be useful for either matching patients to treatment programs, or guiding the differential management of forensic patients to improve treatment compliance.

*Treatment progress.* Chapter 6 describes a study on the relationship between psychopathy and change in dynamic risk factors during treatment of male forensic psychiatric patients. The findings indicated that upon admission, psychopathy was significantly related to more disturbance on a number of dynamic risk indicators. However, psychopathy was *not* found to be significantly related to change scores on indices of anger, egocentrism, impulsivity, lack of insight, negative attitudes, and stress tolerance.

Psychopathic patients did show the expected pattern of treatment noncompliance, compared to nonpsychopaths. It was found that psychopathy was significantly related to a lower level of involvement in treatment activities such as education and work. Factor 2 in particular was negatively associated with treatment involvement.

*Institutional misbehavior.* A significant relationship between PCL-R scores and inpatient disruptive behavior was observed in the studies described in Chapter 5 and Chapter 7. High psychopathy patients were involved in significantly more disruptive incidents. In particular, verbal aggression and violation of hospital rules were more characteristic of patients with high PCL-R scores than of patients with low PCL-R scores. In general, these findings are in line with earlier findings in forensic psychiatric patients supporting the value of the PCL-R as a significant predictor of disruptive behavior in forensic inpatients. In our view, treatment and management of this patient group should be particularly focused on their impulsivity, lack of behavioral control and sensation seeking tendencies.

*Recidivism.* Perhaps most importantly, it was found that rapists scoring high on the PCL-R (i.e., $\geq 26$) were more likely than other rapists to be reconvicted for a sexual, violent nonsexual or general offense (Chapter 7). Survival analyses provided considerable evidence that psychopathic rapists *with deviant sexual preferences* are at much greater risk of committing new sexual offenses than psychopathic offenders without deviant preferences or nonpsychopathic offenders with or without sexual deviance. It is concluded that any comprehensive risk assessment of sex offenders under the TBS-order should consider the combination of psychopathy and sexual deviance.

## PSYCHOPATHY, TREATMENT AND CHANGE

It makes theoretical sense to presume that psychopathic patients are difficult to treat with psychological interventions. Psychopaths, by definition, experience little distress (remorse, guilt, anxiety) that might motivate them for treatment. They see little wrong with themselves, they lack insight, do not empathize with the possible adverse consequences of their behavior for others, and they habitually manipulate other people to achieve their own ends. These characteristics are generally the opposite of those that have been found to be important for effecting positive therapeutic change (e.g., Hemphill & Hart, 2002).

Do our findings justify the conclusion that (PCL-R) psychopaths are 'untreatable'? The answer to this question is a simple 'no', because there is an absence of good evidence. The principal limitation of the empirical literature on the treatment of psychopathic patients to date is that a treatment approach specifically developed for psychopathic patients has not yet been implemented and evaluated (Lösel, 1998). Before (see Chapter 6), we argued that a treatment program based on the principles of risk, need and responsivity, focusing on reducing the risk of violence and destructiveness by modifying the cognitions and behaviors that directly precipitate violent behavior, may maximize change. Subsequently, we argued that the standard of service delivery at the Dr. Henri van der Hoeven Kliniek could be increased by forming homogenous subgroups of patients allowing the development of specialized wards to target the needs of different groups of patients, with the specificity of each ward being based on both patients' treatment needs and security requirements. As a *standard procedure*, criminogenic needs identified during baseline assessment should become treatment targets, and for each target an explicit treatment plan needs to specify how change is to be accomplished. Appropriate interventions delivered in this manner may produce favorable results in the treatment of this high risk group of offenders. Dolan and Coid (1993) mentioned that the 'untreatability' of psychopathic patients may, in part, result from professionals' inadequate assessment of the disorder, followed by a failure to develop, describe and study theoretically sound treatment strategies. Methodologically sound studies would include large groups of clearly defined psychopathic patients, who receive well-designed treatments that are delivered consistently and evaluated systematically with long follow-up periods, using different measures of treatment outcome. In our opinion, and that of others (e.g., Hemphill & Hart, 2002), it seems ethically unjust to deny psychopathic (TBS) patients access to treatment programs on the grounds that they are untreatable. Instead, high priority should be given to designing, implementing, and evaluating treatment programs for these patients (Hildebrand, de Ruiter, & de Vogel, 2003).

## MOTIVATING (PSYCHOPATHIC) PATIENTS TO CHANGE

Offenders required to undergo treatment by legal compulsion are particularly likely to show resistance. Strategies for motivating them to change are deemed appropriate. What motivates (psychopathic) offenders to change?

Motivation for therapy is a multifaceted concept whose parameters are imprecisely defined. Matters relating to motivation to change have been the subject of considerable research in the treatment of addictions, and many addiction concepts and treatment approaches have been adapted for the treatment of offenders. Drawing upon conceptual and empirical frameworks (e.g., Prochaska, DiClemente, & Norcross, 1992; Rosenbaum & Horowitz, 1983) concerning motivation for therapy, Hemphill and Hart (2002) identified various important conditions for change to occur in (forensic) treatment. Acknowledging personal problems and participating in treatment, interest in changing, viewing problems as psychologically-based and believing that interventions could be beneficial, willingness to accept help and to establish a positive relationship with a therapist, striving for autonomy and independence, having clear and realistic treatment goals, and experiencing marked emotional distress, guilt, or shame regarding problems, are strong motivating agents.

According to Wong (2000), the Transtheoretical Model (TM) of change (Prochaska & DiClemente, 1986; Prochaska et al., 1992) may provide a useful heuristic towards a better understanding of how clinicians could provide (psychopathic) offenders with the appropriate treatment at the appropriate time as they progress through the change process. The TM was based on empirical identification of the common features and processes associated with change, and was originally developed in an attempt to explain change in addictive behaviors. Later, it has been expanded into the area of psychological and medical interventions for other disorders (e.g., phobias and depression) for both adults and adolescents (e.g., Belding, Iguchi, & Lamb, 1996; Hemphill & Howell, 2000; Miller & Tonigan, 1996). The TM provides a framework to understand readiness for and commitment to psychological change. The model postulates that individuals who modify their problem behavior move through a series of stages before attaining an identified goal (DiClemente, McConnaughy, Norcross, & Prochaska, 1986; Miller & Rollnick, 1991), including the pre-contemplation, contemplation, preparation, action and maintenance stages. Each stage is characterized by specific patient behaviors. Treatment interventions that are effective for one stage may be ineffective (or even damaging) when applied to the same patient at other stages. Before being successfully treated, the patient may cycle through most or all of the stages more than one time. Relapse or cycling through the stages is considered to be the rule rather than an exception (Prochaska et al., 1992). Change is not considered possible until the patient moves beyond the pre-contemplation stage (i.e., not accepting that a problem exists) and the contemplation stage (uncertainty whether or not change is possible or necessary). Acceptance that a problem exists, and taking responsibility for past and present actions, may, for the (forensic) patient, be the most important step towards progress, facilitating all subsequent efforts in the direction of change. However, insight into the need to change is not in itself sufficient to produce or maintain change.

*Motivational strengths.* Do psychopathic patients have motivational strengths? Hemphill and Hart (2002) suggest psychopathic offenders may have at least four motivational strengths that may help them in therapy: (1) a strong status orientation, (2) a strong desire for and tolerance of novelty, (3) good interpersonal skills, and (4) a desire to be in control. In their opinion, to enhance the motivation of psychopaths, treatment programs should formally assess motivation to participate in treatment, highlight the view that leading a criminal lifestyle is low status, explain the rationale behind psychological interventions, explore their own contributions to personal problems, establish a non-threatening, positive therapeutic alliance with the therapist, emphasize self-sufficiency, attempt to manage antisocial behavior in stead of changing personality structure, focus on cognitive strengths rather than on affective problems, and teach them a variety of therapeutic strategies to change their behavior and maintain positive changes.

## LIMITATIONS OF THE PRESENT RESEARCH

Several (methodological) limitations to the current research deserve attention. First, the treatment program in the hospital where this research was conducted was not specifically designed to address criminogenic needs of adult forensic psychiatric patients. Second, the sample(s) existed by convenience, and experimental manipulation and control could not be conducted.

Another limitation concerns the fact that data collection was restricted to only one forensic hospital. Therefore, caution is warranted regarding the generalizability of the findings. However, in our view, the current stage of development of theory and practice justified this kind of study. Also, we have no reason to believe that the samples we used in our studies were fundamentally different from those of other Dutch forensic institutions. In fact, we consider our sample(s) representative for Dutch offenders with a tbs-order, because they are largely similar in demographic, psychiatric and criminal characteristics (van Emmerik & Brouwers, 2001; de Ruiter, 2003). However, future research involving different, preferably larger (forensic) samples is recommended.

Fourth, of particular concern are the relatively small sample sizes of the different studies reported here, which may have affected the results of the data analyses. The different studies reported in this study all included a total of ± 90 - 95 male patients, and the group classifications that were formed on the basis of the PCL-R total scores contained significantly fewer participants. Larger samples would have resulted in increased power. However, as stated before, this is considered a relatively minor problem given that there is such a paucity of research on the role of the PCL-R in the treatment of Dutch forensic psychiatric patients. Indeed, no prior study has examined the predictive validity of the PCL-R among Dutch forensic patients.

## DIRECTIONS FOR FUTURE RESEARCH

The current study suggests several avenues for future research. Here, we consider several important areas that, in our view, should be research priorities in Dutch forensic psychiatry.

### TEMPORAL STABILITY

Psychopathy is presumed to surface early in life and to remain stable across the lifespan. A corollary of this is that PCL-R scores should demonstrate high test-retest reliability over long time spans. Moreover, individuals identified with psychopathic traits early in life should be the same individuals as those identified with psychopathic traits later in life. This line of research is important for both conceptual and practical reasons. From a conceptual point of view, the stability of PCL-R scores supports the view that psychopathy reflects a stable constellation of personality and behavioral characteristics. The PCL-R is expected to show high test-retest reliability because of the emphasis during assessment on lifetime functioning across several domains. The stability of the PCL-R is suggested by the finding that it consistently is among the most powerful risk factors for antisocial and violent behavior (Harris, Rice, & Quinsey, 1993; Steadman et al., 2000), and that the PCL-R score is a significant predictor of future criminal behavior with long (i.e., $\geq$ 10 years) follow-up periods, and in different samples (e.g., Hemphill, Templeman, Wong, & Hare, 1998; Hildebrand, de Ruiter, & de Vogel, 2004; Rice, Harris, & Cormier, 1992). However, little research has been conducted to investigate the test-retest reliability of the PCL-R. Schroeder, Schroeder, and Hare (1983) were the first to examine the test-retest reliability, using the original 22-item PCL. They conducted a study, using a sample of 42 inmates, with a test-retest interval of approximately 10 months, and obtained a generalizability coefficient of .89.

Rutherford, Cacciola, Alterman, McKay, and Cook (1999) examined the two-year test-retest reliability of the PCL-R in male ($n$ = 200) and female ($n$ = 25) methadone patients. Stability of the PCL-R was reasonably good, whether it was  evaluated as a dichotomous or dimensional measure. Utilizing a diagnostic cutoff score of 25 or more the intraclass correlation coefficients (ICCs) were .48 for men and .67 for women. For the PCL-R total score ICCs were .60 and .65 for men and women, respectively (Rutherford et al., 1999). According to Andrews and Bonta (2003), however, viewing psychopathy as a stable personality trait that changes little over time may be a mistake because there is no *a priori* reason to assume that re-administration of the PCL-R following appropriate treatment would not produce changes in scores. Andrews and Bonta (2003) further argue that the assumption that psychopathy is immutable has diverted researchers from studying the dynamic possibilities of the PCL-R.

## APPLICABILITY OF REVISED MODELS OF (PCL-R) PSYCHOPATHY

At the time we started our research, PCL-R psychopathy was generally believed to be a two-factor construct. However, the results of recent empirical investigations suggest that psychopathy may be composed of three (Cooke, & Michie, 2001) or even four factors

(Hervé & Hare, 2002). In essence, the three-factor model posits that a 13-item PCL-R assesses the superordinate factor of psychopathy, which is underpinned by the three factors *Arrogant and Deceitful Interpersonal Style* (items 1, 2, 4, and 5), *Deficient Emotional Experience* (items 6, 7, 8, and 16), and *Impulsive and Irresponsible Behavioral Style* (items 3, 9, 13, 14, and 15). Compared with the traditional two-factor model, the three-factor model of psychopathy places less emphasis on antisocial/criminal behavior; is more weakly associated with nonspecific indices of social deviance; and, more importantly, appears to better fit data on forensic patients (Cooke & Michie, 2001). Skeem, Mulvey, and Grisso (2003) independently cross-validated the new three-factor model in a large sample ($N$ = 870) of civil psychiatric patients, using the Screening Version of the PCL. They concluded that "Cooke and Michie's (2001) three-factor model of psychopathy is more plausible than the traditional PCL two-factor model with these patients because it better describes the structure of the PCL:SV and more specifically assesses personality deviation" (p. 51). Using these recently-developed factor models may yield important information about the robustness of these factors in diverse populations. However, new research is needed to determine whether the revised factors are anchored in theoretically consistent ways to a broad range of key psychophysiological, clinical, personality, and other variables. For example, does Cooke and Michie's (2001) *Deficient Emotional Experience* factor relate uniquely to deficits in emotional processing? Does it correspond more closely than the *Arrogant and Deceitful Interpersonal Style* or the *Impulsive and Irresponsible Behavioral Style* factor with observational ratings of detached, unempathic interpersonal behavior? In a related vein, future research could also examine whether or not the revised factors are differential predictors of reoffending (i.e., sexual, violent non-sexual, general). For example, does the *Impulsive and Irresponsible Behavioral Style* factor better predict sexual recidivism in rapists, than the *Arrogant and Deceitful Interpersonal Style* factor? This kind of research may lead to the discovery of meaningful subtypes of psychopathy, possibly also with specific neurobiological correlates (see Blair, 2003).

## COMPARATIVE AND INCREMENTAL VALIDITY

In applied settings, it is often useful to examine the unique and shared contributions that psychopathy and other risk factors make to the clinical task at hand. In the area of recidivism research, for example, researchers may want to investigate not only the predictive validity of the PCL-R, but also the additional contribution, if any, that the PCL-R makes to the prediction of (different types of) recidivism beyond that offered by other variables (e.g., number prior convictions) or simple actuarial instruments, such as the Static-99 (Hanson & Thornton, 1999), an actuarial sex offender risk scale. For example, by using multivariate analyses (e.g., binomial logistic regression) researchers may estimate which measure contributes uniquely to the prediction of violence, taking the other measures into account. By building a literature that examines the incremental validity of different measures, clinicians will be in a better position to identify the unique and shared contributions of different variables/measures and to select measures that each contribute unique information to the clinical task.

## TREATMENT PROGRESS AND OUTCOME

*Methodological issues.* Research which evaluates the efficacy of treatment for psychopathy is clearly a priority. Virtually no methodologically sound treatment study has been conducted to evaluate the effectiveness of a contemporary treatment program for psychopaths (see Chapter 6). Such a study would include a large sample of clearly defined psychopathic patients (i.e., assessments made by raters who have the requisite and experience), who have received state of the art treatment interventions that have been delivered consistently and evaluated systematically across long-follow-up periods, using multimodal measures of treatment outcome. We agree with Hemphill and Hart (2002) that although research methodologies have improved greatly over the years, there is still considerable room for improvement for studies that investigate the efficacy of treatment among psychopathic patients.

*Measurement refinement.* Future research should also seek to refine measures' sensitivity to change. The majority of the measures used to assess change in dynamic risk factors during inpatient treatment demonstrated no change (see Chapter 6). Although it is possible that these traits truly did not change during the course of treatment, it is also possible that the measures themselves were not sensitive to change.

*Risk, need, responsivity.* One explanation for our findings (Chapter 6) that patients did not improve on dynamic risk factors is that it may be that the treatment program provided at the hospital deserves review and alteration. We argued that alteration of the treatment program into a multimodal cognitive-behavioral program, based on the principles of risk, need and responsivity, may increase the likelihood of actual change. It may be that the standard of service delivery could be increased by forming homogenous groups of patients and allowing the development of specialized wards to target the needs of different groups of patients (Müller-Isberner, 1993; Rice, Harris, Quinsey, & Cyr, 1990; see also Chapter 7). The treatment program of each ward would then be based on both patient's treatment needs and security requirements. In our view, implementation of a policy of specialization would encourage professional development of therapeutic methods inside the hospital.

*Protective factors.* Why do some psychopathic offenders recidivate while others (seemingly) do not? As yet, there are no definite answers to this important question, however, several researchers have speculated that the presence of various protective, or resiliency, factors may play a significant role in abstinence from further criminal offending (e.g., Grisso, 1998; Hoge & Andrews, 1996; Hoge,  Andrews, & Leschied, 1996; Levenson, Kiehl, & Fitzpatrick, 1995). In this context, protective factors are generally defined as factors that may be responsible for keeping some individuals, who may otherwise be at high risk for engaging in violent or antisocial behavior, from reoffending. Much of the research regarding protective factors has been conducted with juvenile offenders (e.g., Hoge & Andrews, 1996). The purpose of this research is primarily to identify high-risk juveniles and predict which juveniles are most likely to engage in antisocial behavior, usually through an examination of risk or causal factors. As a result of this research, scholars have identified several potential protective factors. Protective factors include biological, psychosocial, and social variables (e.g., Carson & Butcher, 1992). Results from relatively recent studies suggest that a wide variety of variables, related to a number of different psychosocial domains, may act as protective factors: positive family relations, intelligence/education, employment, high self-esteem, absence of a psychiatric history, positive peer  relations, and participation in an organized religion (e.g., Grisso, 1998; Melton, Petrila, Poythress, & Slobogin, 1997; Monahan et al., 2001; Plutchik, 1995). Research suggests that the more protective factors an individual has, the less likely it is that the individual will engage in serious antisocial behavior (Grisso, 1998).

Several scholars have specifically addressed the question why some psychopaths, including noninstitutionalized psychopathic individuals, do not engage in antisocial behavior (e.g., Levenson et al., 1995; Rogers et al., 2000). It may be useful for future research to systematically assess (1) the presence and (2) perceived impact of protective factors after the PCL-R interview is completed[1], especially in relation to treatment outcome and possible reoffending.

In addition, we are particularly in need of studies that closely monitor patients over time, so that we can identify important dynamic risk factors. For example, determining what dynamic factors are most relevant during the early phases of release versus those that do not become important until the TBS-patient's life has stabilized would yield substantial operational gains.

*Impact of motivation.* While many authors propose a link between patient motivation, or willingness to engage in treatment, and treatment success (e.g., Hanson, 2000; Mann, 2000; Mann & Rolnick, 1996; Serin & Kennedy, 1997), little empirical evidence exists substantiating this relationship. Motivation is best understood as a dynamic state. This allows a conceptualization of motivation as a responsivity factor that can be positively influenced to enhance treatment effectiveness. The underlying rationale for the study of motivation is that individuals who are not motivated to actively participate in treatment generally appear to make less progress in intermediate treatment targets and ultimately have greater recidivism rates. For example, Stewart and Millson (1995) identified motivation as a significant factor predicting release outcome. They found that level of motivation was directly related to rates of reoffense. A useful line of future research would be to investigate the applicability of the transtheoretical model of change (described above) in conceptualizing and evaluating patient motivation for treatment.[2] Confirming motivation as a relevant responsivity factor would be an important contribution to the (Dutch) forensic treatment literature since there is now substantial

---

[1] Of course, it would be preferable to use an empirically-validated measure specifically designed to measure the presence of protective factors . To the best of our knowledge, no such instrument is currently available. However, de Vogel, de Ruiter, and Bouman (2003)recently introduced a checklist of 17 protective factors for (sexually) violent behavior that can be used for research purposes in forensic clinical practice in combination with the HCR-20 and/or SVR-20.

[2] Note that the stage of change model is only one of many models that could be employed.

evidence in the general psychotherapy literature that motivation itself can be positively influenced (e.g., McConnaughy, 1987; Miller & Rollnick, 1991).

## PSYCHOPATHIC TRAITS IN CHILDREN AND ADOLESCENTS

Future research in Dutch forensic psychiatry should also investigate psychopathic symptoms in children and adolescents. Although the assessment of psychopathic traits in children and adolescents remains controversial (Edens, Skeem, Cruise, & Kaufman, 2001; Frick, 1998, 2002; Hart, Watt, & Vincent, 2002, Lynam, 2002; Seagrave & Grisso, 2002), there are reasonable grounds to believe that it is possible to assess childhood traits that are similar to psychopathy in adulthood (e.g., Forth & Burke, 1998; Forth, Hart, & Hare, 1990).

The presence of psychopathic symptoms in adolescents has been confirmed (Forth et al., 1990; Mailloux, Forth, & Kroner, 1997; Smith, Gacono, & Kaufman, 1997). Studies have begun to develop evidence for the construct validity of measures — such as the Psychopathy Checklist: Youth Version (PCL:YV; Forth, Kosson, & Hare, in press) — to assess psychopathic traits in adolescents (e.g., Brandt, Kennedy, Patrick, & Curtin, 1997; Chandler & Moran, 1990; Forth et al., 1990; Kosson, Cyterski, Steuerwald, Neumann, & Walker-Matthews, 2002). The psychometric properties of the PCL:YV closely correspond to those of the adult PCL-R (Forth et al., 1990; Harpur & Hare, 1994). Furthermore, the PCL:YV has exhibited reasonably strong predictive validity for violent recidivism in forensic samples of adolescents (e.g., Forth et al., 1990; Gretton, McBride, Hare, O'Shaughnessy, & Kumka, 2001; Harpur & Hare, 1994; Kosson et al., 2002; O'Neill, Lidz, & Heilbrun, 2003). However, a clear demonstration from longitudinal research is needed to prove that psychopathic symptoms in children/adolescents persist into adulthood. It may be that psychopathy-related traits disappear by adulthood as a result of maturation or other factors; it is also possible that these traits emerge in early adulthood in some individuals. To put it differently: Which adolescents are true positives (youth with life course persistent antisocial conduct who will mature into adult psychopathic individuals) and which are false positives (youth who appear antisocial during a developmental phase of adolescence but will adapt in less antisocial ways as they mature; see Moffitt, 1993). If it turns out that it is possible to identify children or adolescents on a developmental trajectory toward adult psychopathy, then perhaps it will be possible to develop early intervention programs that prevent or reduce psychopathic symptoms (e.g., Frick & Ellis, 1999; Gresham, Lane, & Lambros, 2000). Potential ethical problems with this development should be closely monitored (Edens et al., 2001; Ogloff & Lyon, 1998).

## FINAL REMARKS

In many jurisdictions, PCL-R psychopathy now plays an important role in procedures for the prediction of recidivism, violence and response to treatment (e.g., Hare, 1998c). In fact, psychopathy is recognized as a critical factor in violence risk assessment (Hart, 1998), affecting decisions involving parole from prison, access to treatment, and detention under dangerous offender legislation (e.g., Hart, 2001; Lyon & Ogloff, 2000; Zinger & Forth, 1998). Accordingly, the assessment of psychopathy needs to be a fundamental skill for the clinical-forensic psychologist. Although this point seems obvious, particularly in forensic contexts where important psycholegal decisions are made and lives may be greatly affected, Hare (1998c) has amply documented a number of disconcerting examples concerning the misuse of the PCL-R, including (1) mental health professionals using PCL-R assessments based on clinical opinions in stead of the scoring criteria for the items, (2) biased — intentional or otherwise — ratings, and (3) judges "playing psychiatrist" (p. 111). The expert who brings the concept of (PCL-R) psychopathy into the courtroom carries with him a host of ethical and professional issues. Clearly, he needs to have a thorough understanding of the disorder (e.g., prevalence, symptomatology, and implications of the disorder) and appropriate training. Additionally, the expert must maintain his expertise by keeping abreast of new research findings and developments. This is particularly true of psychopathy, which has become the subject of intense empirical investigation over the last decade.

The PCL-R provides researchers and clinicians with a reliable and valid operational measure of a construct that has direct implications for the mental health and criminal justice system (e.g., Chapter 7). What this means for the law is that while psychopaths are more likely than nonpsychopaths to be violent, to recidivate violently, and to cause problems in the institutions in which they are incarcerated or treated, it likely never will be entirely satisfactory for the law. This is because in an individual case, the law does not concern itself with how most people with similar PCL-R scores behave, but, rather, with how the particular individual in question will behave.[3]

According to Hart (1998), the comprehensiveness of a forensic assessment is in doubt *where the legal issue relates to (violence) risk but (PCL-R) psychopathy has not been considered*. In these situations, experts who are unable to provide a strong justification for not considering psychopathy may not be fulfilling professional standards. However, psychopathy must never become *the only* consideration.

---

[3] A fundamental difference between psychology — indeed with science — and law is that science deals with normative data while the law deals with individual cases. This is why researchers are so concerned with sample size and replication, and why statutes are written in an intentionally vague manner, creating a lot of liberty in applying the law to the individual case.

# SUMMARY

The main objective of the research presented in this thesis was to examine the role of PCL-R psychopathy in the treatment of Dutch male forensic psychiatric patients involuntarily admitted to the Dr. Henri van der Hoeven Kliniek, a forensic psychiatric hospital in the Netherlands.

**Chapter 1** offers an introduction to the subsequent chapters. First, we discuss the historical conceptualization of psychopathy as a clinical syndrome. Despite the fact that the concept of psychopathy has been obscured by a multitude of definitions, the clinical description of psychopathy provided by Cleckley (1941), reflecting both the affective and interpersonal characteristics that have traditionally been considered central to psychopathy, including egocentricity, failure to form close emotional bonds, callousness, and lack of guilt, has received widespread acceptance among contemporary researchers and clinicians.

Because traditional assessment procedures, including those based on clinical diagnosis and on self-report inventories, lacked demonstrated reliability and validity, Hare and his colleagues, expanding on Cleckley's conceptualization of psychopathy, and adding items related to antisocial behavior, developed a research tool for operationalizing the construct psychopathy — the 20-item Psychopathy Checklist-Revised (PCL-R; Hare, 1991). At least initially, factor analytic studies of the PCL-R showed that the PCL-R is composed of two distinct and moderately correlated factors. Factor 1 consists of a cluster of eight items reflecting the affective and interpersonal features (core personality traits) of psychopathy, and has been labeled "Selfish, callous and remorseless use of others". Factor 2 consists of nine items reflecting the social deviance features of psychopathy and has been labeled "Chronically unstable and antisocial lifestyle" (Hare, 1991). The remaining three items of the PCL-R did not load on either factor. Recently, however, several authors have suggested that a *three*-factor model that only uses the 13 items of the PCL-R that deal with personality traits (rather than delinquency and social deviance) might actually provide a better fit than the traditional two-factor model (Cooke & Michie, 2001; see also Skeem, Mulvey, & Grisso, 2003).

Each of the PCL-R items is scored on a 3-point ordinal scale (0 = *item does not apply*, 1 = *item applies to a certain extent*, 2 = *item definitely applies*), according to the scoring criteria contained in the PCL-R administration and scoring manual (Hare, 1991). Examiners should score each of the 20 PCL-R items on the basis of the individual's lifetime functioning. The total score can range from 0 to 40, reflecting the degree to which an individual resembles the prototypical psychopath. Hare (1991) suggested a cutoff score of 30 or more to assign a clinical diagnosis of psychopathy. In European research, however, a cutoff score of 26 is often used. Therefore, in our studies, we also used a cutoff of 26 to assign a clinical diagnosis of psychopathy (see Chapters 3-7).

The PCL-R has been rapidly adopted by numerous researchers and clinicians as the gold standard in psychopathy assessment. We review research examining the validity of the PCL-R in terms of covariation with psychological measures and psychophysiological processes. Empirical studies provides evidence that psychopathic individuals show a variety of neurocognitive abnormalities. Studies have uncovered impairments in fear conditioning, startle reflex priming, response modulation, linguistic processing, and autonomic responding to distress cues. Currently, psychopathy is linked to dysfunctioning in the amygdala and the orbitofrontal cortex.

The PCL-R has utility in the prediction of institutional misbehavior in residential settings in a variety of samples of adult male prisoners and forensic psychiatric patients. Moreover, in general, those who score high on the PCL-R show a distinctly negative response to treatment. Finally, research studies generally found that the PCL-R consistently predicts different types (i.e., sexual, violent, general) of recidivism across various clinical settings and samples, including male prison inmates, forensic psychiatric patients and adolescent (sex) offenders. The robust association between PCL-R psychopathy and future violence is evident even after controlling for traditional risk factors that may confound the relationship (e.g., criminal history and/or demographic characteristics).

Next, the main research questions addressed in this thesis are outlined, and the setting where the research was conducted, the Dr. Henri van der Hoeven Kliniek in Utrecht, the Netherlands, is described in some detail — with special reference to psychological assessment procedures used to periodically evaluate treatment progress.

In **Chapter 2**, we describe a special provision in the Dutch criminal code that allows for a period of treatment (custodial care) following a prison sentence for mentally disordered offenders: *Terbeschikkingstelling* (TBS-order), which can be translated as 'disposal to be treated on behalf of the state'. The purpose of TBS is to protect society from unacceptably high risks of recidivism, directly through involuntary admission to a forensic psychiatric hospital, and indirectly through the treatment provided there. Theoretically, treatment under the TBS-order is of indefinite duration if the offender continues to pose a risk to society. Every one or two years the court re-evaluates the patient in order to determine whether the risk of (violent) recidivism is still too high and treatment needs to be continued.

In **Chapters 3-7** empirical studies are described. **Chapter 3** concerns a study examining the reliability and factor structure of the Dutch language version of the PCL-R. In addition, the potential role of two different information sources for scoring the PCL-R, real-life interview versus videotaped interview, was evaluated. Results indicated that the interrater reliability of individual items and of the PCL-R total score was good to excellent. Good agreement on the categorical diagnosis of psychopathy was also obtained (weighted Cohen's $\kappa$ = .63 for simultaneous comparison of three raters). The internal consistency of the PCL-R was high, as indicated by a Cronbach's alpha of 0.87, with an alpha of 0.83 for both Factor 1 and Factor 2. Comparisons between real-life and videotaped interview demonstrated that the information source did not influence the raters' coding. Confirmatory factor analysis (CFA) indicated that the two-factor structure obtained by Hare (1991) in the standardization samples did not fit the current data well. CFA also failed to confirm the three-factor model identified by Cooke and Michie (2001). Exploratory principal components analysis using oblique rotation extracted two main factors, which accounted for 44% of the variance. It is concluded that the Dutch language version of the PCL-R can be reliably rated by trained professionals, its factor structure resembles the traditional two-factor model to some extent, and future research should include larger samples of different populations such as prisoners and general psychiatric patients.

In **Chapter 4**, the association between PCL-R psychopathy and mental disorders defined according to the fourth edition of the *Diagnostic and Statistical Manual of Mental Disorders* (DSM-IV) was examined. Axis I diagnoses were lifetime diagnoses based on consensus between four independent raters. The Structured Interview for DSM-IV

Disorders of Personality (SIDP-IV) was used for the assessment of Axis II disorders. The overall psychiatric morbidity in the sample was high; co-morbidity was the rule, regardless of the degree of PCL-R psychopathy. Psychopathy was significantly positively related to non-alcohol substance use disorders, antisocial and other Cluster B personality disorder (PD). Eighty-eight percent of patients with a PCL-R score $\geq 26$ had a DSM-IV antisocial PD; the reverse was not true. PCL-R scores were also positively correlated with dimensional scores of paranoid, borderline, and narcissistic PD, and with conduct disorder ($< 15$ years) and antisocial behavior since age 15. In general, results are consistent with previous research, providing further evidence for the cross-cultural stability of the PCL-R.

The purpose of the research described in **Chapter 5** was to study the predictive validity of the PCL-R by examining the relationship between PCL-R scores and various types of institutional misbehavior. From daily hospital information bulletins, incidents of verbal abuse, verbal threat, physical violence and violation of hospital rules were derived. Also, the number of seclusion episodes was recorded. Significant correlations were found between PCL-R scores and verbal abuse, verbal threat, violation of rules, total number of incidents, and frequency of seclusion. Psychopaths (PCL-R $\geq 26$) were significantly more often involved in incidents than nonpsychopaths. Multiple regression analyses revealed that the PCL-R Factor 2 score in particular contributed uniquely to the prediction of the total number of incidents. Administration of the PCL-R at admission may enable hospital staff to make appropriate initial placements with respect to treatment needs as well as disruptive potential; PCL-R psychopaths undermine the treatment milieu, specifically through verbal aggression and violation of hospital rules, and treatment and management of this patient group should focus on their impulsivity, lack of behavioral control and sensation seeking tendency.

The main objective of the study presented in **Chapter 6** was to measure treatment outcome by change in indices of dynamic risk factors (i.e., impulsivity, lack of insight, anger, egocentrism, stress tolerance, negative attitudes). It was hypothesized that patients identified as psychopathic would score more unfavorable on indicators of dynamic risk than nonpsychopathic offenders, upon admission to the hospital. In addition, psychopathic patients were expected to show more limited improvement after 20 months of inpatient treatment than nonpsychopathic offenders. Also, the relationship between psychopathy and treatment compliance, as indicated by the attendance rate of therapeutic activities, was investigated. Results indicated that the total patient sample showed limited improvement on indicators of dynamic risk, using different assessment techniques. Psychopathy (PCL-R score $\geq$ 26) was significantly related to pathology on a limited number of indicators of dynamic risk. Contrary to our hypothesis, psychopathy was *not* found to be significantly related to change scores on any of the indicators of dynamic risk. However, psychopaths did show the expected pattern of treatment noncompliance, compared to nonpsychopaths. Psychopathy was significantly associated with a lower level of involvement in treatment activities such as education and work. Especially Factor 2 was negatively associated with treatment involvement. It is argued that lack of progress should not be too easily attributed to psychopathy, and psychopathic patients should not be excluded from forensic inpatient treatment in advance.

In **Chapter 7**, the role of psychopathy and sexual deviance in predicting recidivism in a sample of 94 rapists involuntarily admitted to the Dr. Henri van der Hoeven Kliniek between 1975 and 1996, was investigated. The predictive utility of grouping offenders based on combinations of psychopathy and sexual deviance was also investigated. Furthermore, we explored the relationship between PCL-R scores and serious institutional misbehavior (i.e., unauthorized absence, physical violence, alcohol/drug use, and episodes of seclusion). Base rates for sexual, violent nonsexual, violent (including sexual) and general recidivism were 34%, 47%, 54%, and 71%, respectively. Receiver Operating Characteristic (ROC) analyses provided moderate to strong support for the predictive validity of the PCL-R for inpatient disruptive behavior and recidivism outcomes. Patients scoring high on the PCL-R ($\geq$ 26) were more likely than other patients to be reconvicted for a sexual, violent nonsexual or general offense. Survival analyses provided strong evidence that psychopathic rapists with deviant sexual preferences are at much greater risk of committing new sexual offenses than psychopathic offenders without deviant preferences or nonpsychopathic offenders with or without sexual deviance. It is concluded that not all rapists are equally likely to reoffend, and comprehensive risk assessment should consider the combination of psychopathy and sexual deviance. Further research is needed to determine whether these factors are changeable by treatment.

Chapter 8 concludes the present thesis. The major findings are discussed, a critical analysis of the thesis is presented, recommendations for clinical practice are given, and suggestions for further research on psychopathy are outlined. Finally, some of the concerns about the potential misuse of the PCL-R are briefly discussed.

# SAMENVATTING

In dit proefschrift staat de vraag naar de rol van de diagnose psychopathie in de behandeling van ter beschikking gestelden, die zijn opgenomen in de Dr. Henri van der Hoeven Kliniek — één van de forensisch psychiatrische instituten die ons land kent — centraal.

**Hoofdstuk 1** is een inleiding op de daarop volgende hoofdstukken. Eerst wordt de historische ontwikkeling van het construct psychopathie geschetst. Aan het werk van verschillende auteurs (zie Hildebrand, de Ruiter, & de Vogel, 2003) kunnen de volgende kenmerkende aspecten van de diagnose psychopathie worden ontleend: (1) gebrek aan empathie en het onvermogen een emotionele band met anderen aan te gaan, (2) manipulerend gedrag, bedoeld om de ander te overheersen en te misbruiken, (3) gebrek aan schaamte en schuldgevoel en (4) onbetrouwbaarheid. De psychopaat is goed in staat zichzelf achter een 'masker van gezondheid' te verbergen (Cleckley, 1941). In het contact met anderen toont hij vele gezichten; enerzijds kan hij charmerend, beleefd en sociaal geëngageerd overkomen, anderzijds is hij hard, koud en gevoelloos, of juist agressief en intimiderend. Ook voelt hij goed de zwakheden en emoties van anderen aan en buit deze uit wanneer het hem uitkomt. Daarnaast is er in veel gevallen sprake van chronisch onverantwoordelijk en antisociaal gedrag.

Teneinde de mate van psychopathie betrouwbaar vast te kunnen stellen ontwikkelden Hare en collega's de *Psychopathy Checklist-Revised* (PCL-R; Hare, 1991). De PCL-R bestaat uit 20 items die traditioneel onderverdeeld worden in twee dimensies. Factor 1 ('egoïstisch, ongevoelig en zonder wroeging gebruik maken van anderen') beschrijft een constellatie van acht persoonlijkheidseigenschappen, die volgens de meeste onderzoekers de kern vormen van psychopathie. Factor 2 ('chronisch instabiel en antisociaal gedrag') bestaat uit negen items, die gedragskenmerken bevatten die horen bij een antisociale levensstijl. Deze dimensie vertoont grote overeenkomst met de criteria van de antisociale persoonlijkheidsstoornis, zoals die zijn geformuleerd in de vierde editie van de *Diagnostic and Statistical Manual of Mental Disorders* (DSM-IV; American Psychiatric Association, 1994). Recent zijn echter diverse studies gepubliceerd waaruit blijkt, dat de

items van de PCL-R wellicht beter kunnen worden onderverdeeld in drie factoren (Cooke
& Michie, 2001; Skeem, Mulvey, & Grisso, 2003).

De 20 PCL-R items dienen te worden gescoord op basis van gegevens die
verkregen zijn via de afname van een semi-gestructureerd interview en de analyse van
aanwezige dossierinformatie. De items worden gescoord op een driepuntsschaal ('2' = *item
is van toepassing*; '1' = *item is in een aantal opzichten van toepassing*; '0' = *item is niet
van toepassing*). De PCL-R levert een score op die aangeeft in hoeverre de persoon
volgens de beoordelaar overeenkomt met de 'prototypische psychopaat'. Hare (1991,
1996) adviseert om een kritische waarde van 30 te gebruiken om iemand als psychopaat te
classificeren. In Europees onderzoek wordt echter vaak een *cut-off* score van 26
gehanteerd. In navolging van eerder Europees onderzoek met de PCL-R definieerden wij
psychopathie eveneens als een score van 26 of meer op de PCL-R (zie de hoofdstukken 3
t/m 7).

De PCL-R is in de afgelopen decennia uitgegroeid tot hét standaard meetinstrument
voor het stellen van de diagnose psychopathie. We bespreken de talrijke, veelal Noord-
Amerikaanse, wetenschappelijke studies naar (PCL-R) psychopathie, waarbij in het
bijzonder aandacht wordt besteed aan onderzoek op het gebied van neurobiologische
afwijkingen bij psychopathie, alsmede aan onderzoek naar de voorspellende waarde van de
diagnose psychopathie. De resultaten uit neurobiologisch onderzoek wijzen op de
aanwezigheid van structurele en functionele afwijkingen in een aantal hersengebieden
(amygdala, de hippocampus en prefrontale hersengebieden), welke ten grondslag liggen
aan de gebrekkige gedragsregulatie en deficiënte emotieverwerkingsprocessen bij
psychopathie. De PCL-R score blijkt een krachtige voorspeller van gewelddadige en
seksuele recidive bij diverse groepen delinquenten en forensisch psychiatrische patiënten,
alsmede van een ongunstige behandelrespons en agressieve incidenten (verbale agressie,
fysiek geweld) tijdens detentie of behandeling.

Vervolgens staan we stil bij de onderzoeksvragen die in deze dissertatie onderwerp
van onderzoek zijn en beschrijven we de setting waar de diverse studies zijn uitgevoerd, de
Dr. Henri van der Hoeven Kliniek te Utrecht — met speciale aandacht voor (de
implementatie van het) psychologisch (test)onderzoek teneinde de voortgang van de
behandeling te evalueren.

In **Hoofdstuk 2** wordt in kort bestek de strafrechtelijke maatregel terbeschikkingstelling (tbs) toegelicht. De maatregel tbs is bedoeld voor delinquenten die een ernstig delict hebben gepleegd en daarvoor door de rechter verminderd toerekeningsvatbaar zijn verklaard. Bovendien bestaat er (volgens gedragsdeskundigen) een aanzienlijke kans op recidive met een soortgelijk misdrijf. Bij het opleggen van de maatregel wordt een verband verondersteld tussen de psychische stoornis van de betrokkene en het door hem/haar gepleegde delict. Het doel van de tbs — beveiliging van de maatschappij — wordt op korte termijn gerealiseerd door de vrijheidsbeneming en op langere termijn door een behandeling gericht op structurele gedragsverandering, waartoe de ter beschikking gestelde wordt opgenomen in één van de 13 forensisch psychiatrische instellingen die ons land telt.

In de hoofdstukken 3 t/m 7 worden de empirische studies beschreven. In **Hoofdstuk 3** staan de betrouwbaarheid en factorstructuur van de (Nederlandse versie van de) PCL-R centraal Ook onderzochten wij de potentiële invloed van verschillende informatiebronnen (*life* interviews versus interviews opgenomen op video) op de PCL-R score. De interbeoordelaarsbetrouwbaarheid, vastgesteld door *drie* onafhankelijke beoordelaars per patiënt, was goed tot uitstekend, zowel voor de PCL-R totaalscore als voor de individuele items. Ook was er een goede overeenstemming over de categoriale diagnose psychopathie (Cohen's $\kappa = .63$). De interne consistentie bleek eveneens goed te zijn (Cronbach's $\alpha = .87$ voor de PCL-R totaalscore en .83 voor zowel Factor 1 als Factor 2). Vergelijking van *life* interviews en interviews opgenomen op video bracht aan het licht dat de informatiebron niet van invloed was op de PCL-R score. Confirmatieve factoranalyse gaf (te) weinig steun voor de originele twee-factor structuur van de PCL-R. Ook werd weinig steun gevonden voor de door Cooke en Michie (2001) geïdentificeerde drie-factor structuur. Principale Componenten analyse leverde een twee-factor oplossing die samen 44% van de variantie verklaarde. De bevindingen leveren evidentie voor de betrouwbaarheid van de PCL-R. De factorstructuur vertoonde weliswaar gelijkenis met de originele factor oplossing, toekomstig onderzoek met de PCL-R in Nederland behoeft grotere steekproeven, waaronder gedetineerden en psychiatrische patiënten.

In **Hoofdstuk 4** wordt de relatie onderzocht tussen de PCL-R score en DSM-IV As I en As II stoornissen. As I diagnoses waren *lifetime* diagnoses gebaseerd op het consensus oordeel van vier onafhankelijke beoordelaars. As II diagnoses werden vastgesteld met behulp van het *Structured Interview for DSM-IV Disorders of Personality* (SIDP-IV). Psychopathie bleek significant geassocieerd aan middelenmisbruik (exclusief alcohol), en de antisociale persoonlijkheidsstoornis, alsmede aan andere Cluster B persoonlijkheidsstoornissen. Achtentachtig procent van de patiënten met een PCL-R score ≥ 26 hadden een antisociale persoonlijkheidsstoornis; het omgekeerde was niet het geval. PCL-R scores waren eveneens positief gerelateerd aan dimensionele scores van de paranoïde, borderline, en narcistische persoonlijkheidsstoornis, en met de gedragsstoornis (< 15 jaar) en antisociaal gedrag na het 15$^e$ jaar. De resultaten komen overeen met eerdere onderzoeksbevindingen, hetgeen de cross-culturele stabiliteit van de PCL-R verder ondersteunt.

Wat is de waarde van de PCL-R diagnose psychopathie voor het voorspellen van incidenten (verbale agressie, fysieke bedreiging, overtreding van kliniekregels) tijdens de behandeling? Deze vraag staat centraal in het onderzoek, dat in **Hoofdstuk 5** wordt beschreven. Uit de resultaten komt naar voren dat patiënten die hoog scoren op de PCL-R vaker verbaal agressief zijn, vaker dreigend gedrag vertonen tegen staf en medepatiënten en vaker kliniekregels overtreden dan laagscoorders. Psychopathische patiënten (PCL-R ≥ 26) waren significant vaker betrokken bij dit soort incidenten dan niet-psychopaten. Psychopathische patiënten ondermijnen het behandelklimaat, vooral door verbaal agressief gedrag en het overtreden van kliniekregels. Gesuggereerd wordt in de behandeling van deze categorie patiënten veel aandacht te besteden aan de gebrekkige impulsbeheersing en de neiging tot *sensation seeking*.

De primaire doelstelling van de strafrechtelijke maatregel tbs is het zo goed mogelijk uitbannen van gevaar (risico) voor de samenleving, dat uitgaat van de 'gestoorde' pleger van een ernstig delict. Dit impliceert dat — teneinde het recidiverisico te verminderen — de behandeling in de eerste plaats gericht dient te zijn op afname van *risicofactoren* voor nieuw delictgedrag die in principe veranderbaar zijn, zogenaamde dynamische risicofactoren, zoals impulsiviteit, egocentrisme en hostiliteit. In de studie die in **Hoofdstuk 6** wordt gerapporteerd staat de relatie tussen psychopathie en eventuele veranderingen op indicatoren van dynamische risicofactoren na 20 maanden intramurale behandeling, centraal. De verwachting was (1) dat psychopathische patiënten (PCL-R score ≥ 26) bij opname ongunstiger scoren op indicatoren van dynamische risicofactoren en (2) dat psychopathische patiënten ten opzichte van niet-psychopathische patiënten minder verbetering laten zien op deze indicatoren na 20 maanden behandeling. Uit de studie bleek dat psychopathie inderdaad significant gerelateerd was aan hogere scores op verschillende indicatoren van dynamische risicofactoren. Bij de nameting na gemiddeld 20 maanden bleek echter dat psychopathie *niet* samenhangt met de verschilscores op indices van de risicofactoren hostiliteit, impulsiviteit, egocentriciteit, gebrek aan inzicht, negatieve houding en stresstolerantie. Wél vertoonden psychopaten het verwachte patroon wat betreft *treatment (non)compliance*; psychopathische patiënten verzuimden significant vaker dan niet-psychopaten behandelingsactiviteiten als arbeidstraining en onderwijs. Voor de activiteiten creatieve/expressieve vorming, sport/bewegingsvorming en psychotherapie werden geen significante verschillen gevonden tussen psychopathische en niet-psychopathische patiënten. Gebrek aan vooruitgang in forensisch psychiatrische behandeling dient niet al te snel aan de mate van psychopathie te worden toegeschreven, en psychopathische patiënten dienen niet op voorhand van behandeling te worden uitgesloten.

**Hoofdstuk 7** beschrijft een onderzoek naar de relatie tussen psychopathie, seksuele deviatie en recidive binnen een groep verkrachters/aanranders die tussen 1975 en 1996 in de Dr. Henri van der Hoeven Kliniek werd opgenomen. Op basis van bevindingen uit eerder onderzoek was onze hypothese dat verkrachters/ aanranders met een hoge score op de PCL-R meer recidiveren dan laagscoorders op de PCL-R, ongeacht het type recidive (seksueel, gewelddadig niet-seksueel, enige recidive). Bovendien verwachtten wij dat psychopathische verkrachters met een deviante seksuele voorkeur vaker recidiveren met een *seksueel* delict dan andere typen verkrachters. De eerste hypothese werd bevestigd: de *base rate* voor zowel seksuele als gewelddadige niet-seksuele recidive was significant hoger bij verkrachters met een hoge PCL-R score — in vergelijking met laagscoorders. De tweede hypothese werd eveneens bevestigd. Nieuwe veroordelingen voor een seksueel delict konden weliswaar worden voorspeld door de factoren psychopathie en seksuele deviatie afzonderlijk, maar de resultaten van ons onderzoek geven sterke aanwijzingen dat de aanwezigheid van de specifieke *combinatie* psychopathie en seksuele deviatie een sterk verhoogd risico met zich meebrengt. De resultaten onderstrepen het grote belang van een systematische, empirisch onderbouwde inschatting van het recidiverisico in forensisch diagnostisch onderzoek.

In **Hoofdstuk 8** wordt de slotbalans opgemaakt. Nadat de belangrijkste onderzoeksbevindingen zijn samengevat en bediscussieerd wordt ingegaan op de klinische relevantie van het onderzoek, waarbij de vraag in hoeverre psychopathie te behandelen is, centraal staat. Ook doen wij enige suggesties voor toekomstig onderzoek naar psychopathie. Tenslotte gaan wij kort in op enkele potentiële gevaren die kleven aan het verkeerd gebruik van de PCL-R.

# REFERENCES

Abraham, P., Lepisto, L.B., Lewis, M.G., Schultz, L., & Finelberg, S. (1994). Changes in Rorschach variables of adolescents in residential treatment: An outcome study. *Journal of Personality Assessment, 62*, 505-514.

Alterman, A.I., Cacciola, J.S., & Rutherford, M.J. (1993). Reliability of the Revised Psychopathy Checklist in substance abuse patients. *Psychological Assessment: A Journal of Consulting and Clinical Psychology, 5*, 442-448.

Alterman, A.I., Rutherford, M.J., Cacciola, J.S., McKay, J.R., & Boardman, C.R. (1997). Prediction of 7 months methadone maintenance treatment response by four measures of antisociality. *Drug and Alcohol Dependence, 49*, 217-223.

American Psychiatric Association. (1952). *Diagnostic and statistical manual of mental disorders*. Washington, DC: Author.

American Psychiatric Association. (1968). *Diagnostic and statistical manual of mental disorders* (2nd ed.). Washington, DC: Author.

American Psychiatric Association. (1980). *Diagnostic and statistical manual of mental disorders* (3rd ed.). Washington, DC: Author.

American Psychiatric Association (1987). *Diagnostic and statistical manual of mental disorders* (3rd ed. rev.). Washington, DC: Author.

American Psychiatric Association (1994). *Diagnostic and statistical manual of mental disorders* (4th ed.). Washington, DC: Author.

Andersen, H.S., Sestoft, D., Lillebæk, T., Mortensen, E.L., & Kramp, P. (1999). Psychopathy and psychopathological profiles in prisoners on remand. *Acta Psychiatrica Scandinavica, 99*, 33-39.

Andrews, D.A. (1995). The psychology of criminal conduct and effective treatment. In J. McGuire (Ed.), *What works: Reducing reoffending — Guidelines from research and practice* (pp. 35-62). Chichester, UK: Wiley.

Andrews, D.A., & Bonta, J. (1994). *The psychology of criminal conduct*. Cincinnati, OH: Anderson.

Andrews, D.A., & Bonta, J. (1995). *The Level of Service Inventory – Revised*. Toronto, Ontario, Canada: Multi-Health Systems.

Andrews, D.A., & Bonta, J. (2003). *The psychology of criminal conduct* (3rd ed.). Cincinnati, OH: Anderson.

Andrews, D.A., Bonta, J., & Hoge, R.D. (1990). Classification for effective rehabilitation: Rediscovering psychology. *Criminal Justice and Behavior, 17*, 19-52.

Andrews, D.A., Zinger, I., Hoge, R.D., Bonta, J., Gendreau, P., & Cullen, F.T. (1990). Does correctional treatment work? A clinically relevant and psychologically informed meta-analysis. *Criminology, 28*, 369-404.

Arnett, P.A., Howland, E.W., Smith, S.S., & Newman, J.P. (1993). Autonomic responsivity during passive avoidance in incarcerated psychopaths. *Personality and Individual Differences, 14*, 173-184.

Babiak, P. (1995).When psychopaths go to work: A case study of an industrial psychopath. *Applied Psychology: An International Review, 44*, 171-178.

Babiak, P. (2000). Psychopathic manipulation at work. In C.B. Gacono (Ed.), *The clinical and forensic assessment of psychopathy: A practitioner's guide* (pp. 287-311). Mahwah, NJ: Erlbaum.

Ball, E.M., Young, D., Dotson, L.A., Brothers, L.T., & Robbins, D. (1994). Factors associated with dangerous behavior in forensic inpatients: Results from a pilot study. *Bulletin of the American Academy of Psychiatry and Law, 22*, 605-620.

Barbaree, H.E., Seto, M.C., & Langton, M.C. (2001, November). *Psychopathy, treatment behavior and sex offender recidivism: Extended follow-up.* Paper presented at the 20th Annual Research and Treatment Conference of the Association for the Treatment of Sexual Abusers (ATSA), San Antonio, Texas.

Barbaree, H.E., Seto, M.C., Langton, M.C., & Peacock, E.J. (2001). Evaluating the predictive accuracy of six risk assessment instruments for adult sex offenders. *Criminal Justice and Behavior, 28*, 490-521.

Barbaree, H.E., Seto, M.C., Serin, R.C., Amos, N.L., & Preston, D.L. (1994). Comparison between sexual and nonsexual rapist subtypes. *Criminal Justice and Behavior, 21*, 95-114.

Barratt, E.S. (1994). Impulsiveness and aggression. In J. Monahan & H. Steadman (Eds.), *Violence and mental disorder: Developments in risk assessment* (pp. 61-79). Chicago: University of Chicago Press.

Barron, F. (1953). An ego strength scale which predicts response to psychotherapy. *Journal of Consulting Psychology, 17*, 327-333.

Bechara, A., Damasio, A.R., Damasio, H., & Anderson, S.W. (1994). Intensivity to future consequences following damage to human prefrontal cortex. *Cognition, 50*, 7-15.

Bechara, A., Damasio, H., Damasio, A.R., & Lee, G.P. (1999). Different contributions of the human amygdala and ventromedial prefrontal cortex to decision-making. *Journal of Neuroscience, 18*, 428-437.

Beck, A.T., Freeman, A., & Associates (1990). *Cognitive theory of personality disorders.* New York: Guilford.

Beek, D.J. van (1999). *De delictscenario procedure bij seksueel agressieve delinquenten.* [The offence script procedure with sexually aggressive offenders]. Doctoral dissertation University of Amsterdam. Deventer, the Netherlands: Gouda Quint.

Belding, M.A., Iguchi, M.Y., & Lamb, R.J. (1996). Stages of change in methadone maintenance: Assessing the convergent validity of two measures. *Psychology of Addictive Behaviors, 10*, 157-166.

Belfrage, H., & Douglas, K.S. (2002). Treatment effects on forensic psychiatric patients measured with the HCR-20 violence risk assessment scheme. *International Journal of Forensic Mental Health, 1*, 25-36.

Belfrage, H., Fransson, G., & Strand, S. (2000). Prediction of violence using the HCR-20: A prospective study in two maximum-security correctional institutions. *Journal of Forensic Psychiatry, 11*, 167-175.

Ben-Porath, Y.S. (1990). Cross-cultural assessment of personality: The case for replicatory factor analysis. In J.N. Butcher & C.D. Spielberger (Eds.), *Advances in personality assessment* (Vol. 8, pp. 27-48). Hillsdale, NJ: Erlbaum.

Birnbaum, K. (1914). *Die psychopathischen Verbrecher* (2nd ed.). Leipzig, Germany: Thieme.

Blackburn, R. (1975). An empirical classification of psychopathic personality. *British Journal of Psychiatry, 127*, 456-460.

Blackburn, R. (1986). Patterns of personality deviation among violent offenders: Replication and extension of an empirical taxonomy. *British Journal of Criminology, 26*, 254-269.

Blackburn, R. (1988). On moral judgements and personality disorders: The myth of psychopathic personality revisited. *British Journal of Psychiatry, 153*, 505-512.

Blackburn, R. (1993). Clinical programs with psychopaths. In C.R. Hollin & K. Howells (Eds.), *Clinical approaches to the mentally disordered offender* (pp. 179-208). Chichester, UK: Wiley.

Blackburn, R. (1998a). Psychopathy and personality disorder: Implication of interpersonal theory. In D.J. Cooke, A.E. Forth, & R.D. Hare (Eds.), *Psychopathy: Theory, research and implications for society* (pp. 269-301). Dordrecht, the Netherlands: Kluwer.

Blackburn, R. (1998b). Criminality and the interpersonal circle in mentally disordered offenders. *Criminal Justice and Behavior, 25*, 155-176.

Blackburn, R. (2001). Treatment in high security hospitals. In C.R. Hollin (Ed.), *Handbook of offender assessment and treatment* (pp. 525-535). Chichester, UK: Wiley.

Blackburn, R., Crellin, M.C., Morgan, E.M., & Tulloch, R.M.B. (1990). Prevalence of personality disorders in a special hospital population. *Journal of Forensic Psychiatry, 1*, 43-52.

Blair, R.J.R. (1995). A cognitive developmental approach to morality: Investigating the psychopath. *Cognition, 57*, 1-29.

Blair, R.J.R. (1999). Responsiveness to distress cues in the child with psychopathic tendencies. *Personality and Individual Differences, 22*, 731-739.

Blair, R.J.R. (2001). Neurocognitive models of aggression, the antisocial personality disorders, and psychopathy. *Journal of Neurology, Neurosurgery, and Psychiatry, 71*, 727-731.

Blair, R.J.R. (2003). Neurobiological basis of psychopathy. *British Journal of Psychiatry, 182*, 5-7.

Blair, R.J.R., Colledge, E., & Mitchell, D.G.V. (2001). Somatic markers and response reversal: Is there orbitofrontal cortex dysfunction in boys with psychopathic tendencies? *Journal of Abnormal Child Psychology, 29*, 499-511.

Blair, R.J.R., Jones, R.L., Clark, F., & Smith, M. (1997). The psychopathic individual: A lack of responsiveness to distress cues? *Psychophysiology, 34*, 192-198.

Blair, R.J.R., Mitchell, D.G.V., Richell, R.A., Kelly, S., Leonard, A., Newman, C., & Scott, S.K. (2002). Turning a deaf ear to fear: Impaired recognition of vocal affect in psychopathic individuals. *Journal of Abnormal Psychology, 111*, 682-686.

Blashfield, R.K., & Draguns, J.G. (1976). Evaluative criteria for psychiatric classification. *Journal of Abnormal Psychology, 85*, 140-150.

Bodholt, R.H., Richards, H.R., & Gacono, C.B. (2000). Assessing psychopathy in adults: The Psychopathy Checklist-Revised and Screening Version. In C.B. Gacono (Ed.), *The clinical and forensic assessment of psychopathy: A practitioner's guide* (pp. 55-86). Mahwah, NJ: Erlbaum.

Boer, D.P., Hart, S.D., Kropp, P.R., & Webster, C.D. (1997). *Manual for the Sexual Violence Risk-20: Professional guidelines for assessing risk of sexual violence.* Vancouver, Canada: Institute against Family Violence.

Boer, D.P., Wilson, R.J., Gauthier, C.M., & Hart, S.D. (1997). Assessing risk for sexual violence: Guidelines for clinical practice. In C.D. Webster & M.A. Jackson (Eds.), *Impulsivity: Theory, assessment, and treatment* (pp. 326-342). New York: Guilford.

Bonta, J., & Hanson, R.K. (1994). *Gauging the risk for violence: Measurement, impact and strategies for change.* [User Report No. 1994-09]. Ottawa, Canada: Solicitor General of Canada.

Bonta, J., Harris, A., Zinger, I., & Carriere, D. (1996). *The crown files research project: A study of dangerous offenders.* Ottawa, Canada: Solicitor General of Canada.

Bonta, J., Law, M., & Hanson, K. (1998). The prediction of criminal and violent recidivism among mentally disordered offenders: A meta-analysis. *Psychological Bulletin, 123*, 123-142.

Borum, R. (1996). Improving the clinical practice of violence risk assessment. *American Psychologist, 51*, 945-956.

Brandt, J.R., Kennedy, W.A., Patrick, C.J., & Curtin, J.J. (1997). Assessment of psychopathy in a population of incarcerated adolescent offenders. *Psychological Assessment, 9*, 429-435.

Brink, W. van den, & Jong, C.A.J. de (1992). *De Nederlandse versie van het Structured Interview for DSM-III-R Personality Disorders* [The Dutch version of the

Structured interview for DSM-III-R Personality Disorders]. Eindhoven, the Netherlands: Instituut voor Verslavingszorg Brabant.

Buffington-Vollum, J., Edens, J.F., Johnson, D.W., & Johnson, J.K. (2002). Psychopathy as a predictor of institutional misbehavior among sex offenders: A prospective replication. *Criminal Justice and Behavior, 29*, 497-511.

Bursten, B. (1972). The manipulative personality. *Archives of General Psychiatry, 26*, 318-321.

Bursten, B. (1973). Some narcissistic personality types. *International Journal of Psychoanalysis, 54*, 287-299.

Butcher, J.N., Dahlstrom, W.G., Graham, J.R., Tellegen, A., & Kaemmer, B. (1989). *Minnesota Multiphasic Personality Inventory-2 (MMPI-2): Manual for administration and scoring.* Minneapolis, MN: University of Minnesota Press.

Butcher, J.N., Graham, J.R., Ben-Porath, Y.S., Tellegen, A., & Kaemmer, B. (2001). *MMPI-2: Minnesota Multiphasic Personality Inventory-2 (MMPI-2): Manual for administration, scoring and interpretation.* Minneapolis, MN: University of Minnesota Press.

Butcher, J.N., & Han, K. (1995). Development of an MMPI-2 scale to assess the presentation of self in a superlative manner: The S scale. In J.N. Butcher & C.D. Spielberger (Eds.), *Advances in personality assessment* (pp. 25-50). Hillsdale, NJ: Erlbaum.

Carson, R.C. (1979). Personality and exchange in developing relationships. In R.L. Burgess & T.L. Huston (Eds.), *Social exchange in developing relationships* (pp. 247-269). New York: Academic Press.

Carson, R.C., & Butcher, J.N. (1992). *Abnormal psychology and modern life* (9th ed.). New York: Harper Collins.

Cattell, R.B. (1966). The scree test for the number of factors. *Multivariate Behavioral Research, 1*, 245-276.

Chandler, M., & Moran, T. (1990). Psychopathy and moral development: A comparative study of delinquent and nondelinquent youth. *Development and Psychopathology, 2*, 227-246.

Cleckley, H. (1941). *The mask of sanity.* St. Louis, MO: Mosby.

Cleckley, H. (1982). *The mask of sanity* (6th ed.). St. Louis, MO: Mosby.

Cohen, J. (1980). A coefficient of agreement for nominal scales. *Education and Psychological Measurement, 1*, 37-46.

Cohen, J. (1988). *Statistical power analysis for the behavioral sciences* (2nd ed.). Hillsdale, NJ: Erlbaum.

Coid, J.W. (1992). DSM-III diagnosis in criminal psychopaths: A way forward. *Criminal Behaviour and Mental Health, 2*, 78-94.

Cooke, D.J. (1995). Psychopathic disturbance in the Scottish prison population: The cross-cultural generalizability of the Hare Psychopathy Checklist. *Psychology, Crime, and Law, 2*, 101-108.

Cooke, D.J. (1996). Psychopathic personality in different cultures: What do we know? What do we need to find out? *Journal of Personality Disorders, 10*, 23-40.

Cooke, D.J. (1997). The Barlinnie Special Unit: The rise and fall of a therapeutic experiment. In E. Cullen, L. Jones, & R. Woodward (Eds.), *Therapeutic communities for offenders* (pp. 101-120). New York: Wiley.

Cooke, D.J. (1998). Psychopathy across cultures. In D.J. Cooke, A.E. Forth, & R.D. Hare (Eds.), *Psychopathy: Theory, research, and implications for society* (pp. 13-45). Dordrecht, the Netherlands: Kluwer.

Cooke, D.J., Kosson, D., & Michie, C. (2001). Psychopathy and ethnicity: Structural, item and test generalizability of the Psychopathy Checklist-Revised (PCL-R) in Caucasian and African-American participants. *Psychological Assessment, 13*, 531-542.

Cooke, D.J., & Michie, C. (1997). An item response theory evaluation of Hare's Psychopathy Checklist. *Psychological Assessment, 9*, 2-13.

Cooke, D.J., & Michie, C. (1999). Psychopathy across cultures. *Journal of Abnormal Psychology, 108*, 58-68.

Cooke, D.J., & Michie, C. (2001). Refining the construct of psychopathy: Towards a hierarchical model. *Psychological Assessment, 13*, 171-188.

Cooke, D.J., & Michie, C., Hart, S.D., & Hare, R.D. (1999). Evaluating the Screening Version of the Hare Psychopathy Checklist-Revised: An item response theory analysis. *Psychological Assessment, 11*, 3-13.

Cooke, D. J., & Philip, L. (2001). To treat or not to treat? An empirical perspective. In C.R. Hollin (Ed.), *Handbook of offender assessment and treatment* (pp. 17-34). Chichester, UK: Wiley.

Côté, G., & Hodgins, S. (1992). The prevalence of major mental disorders among homicide offenders. *International Journal of Law and Psychiatry, 15*, 89-99.

Cox, D.R. (1972). Regression models and life tables. *Journal of the Royal Statistical Society, 34*, 187-220.

Craft, M.J. (1965). *Ten studies into psychopathic personality*. Bristol, UK: John Wright.

Cunningham, M.D., & Reidy, T.J. (1998). Antisocial personality disorder and psychopathy: Diagnostic dilemmas in classifying patterns of antisocial behavior in sentencing evaluations. *Behavioural Sciences and the Law, 16*, 333-351.

Darke, S., Kaye, S., Finlay-Jones, R., & Hall, W. (1998). Factor structure of psychopathy among methadone maintenance patients. *Journal of Personality Disorders, 12*, 162-171.

Day, R., & Wong, S. (1996). Anomalous perceptual asymmetries for negative emotional stimuli in the psychopath. *Journal of Abnormal Psychology, 105*, 648-652.

Dernevik, M. (1999, July). *Implementing risk assessment procedures in a forensic psychiatric setting*. Paper presented at the joint conference of the American Psychology-Law Society and the European Association of Psychology and Law. Dublin, Ireland.

Dias, R., Robbins, T.W., & Roberts, A.C. (1996). Dissociation in prefrontal cortex of affective and attentional shifts. *Nature, 380*, 69-72.

DiClemente, C.C. (1999). Motivation for change: Implications for substance abuse treatment. *Psychological Science, 10*, 209-213.

Dolan, B. (1998). Therapeutic community treatment for severe personality disorders. In T. Millon, E. Simonsen, M. Birket-Smith, & R.D. Davis (Eds.), *Psychopathy: Antisocial, criminal, and violent behavior* (pp. 407-430). New York: Guilford.

Dolan, B., & Coid, J. (1993). *Psychopathic and antisocial personality disorders: Treatment and research issues*. London: Gaskell.

Doren, D.M. ( 1987). *Understanding and treating the psychopath*. New York: Wiley.

Doren, D.M. (1998). Recidivism base rates, predictions of sex offender recidivism, and the sexual predator commitment laws. *Behavioral Sciences and the Law*, *16*, 97-114.

Douglas, K.S., Cox, D.N., & Webster, C.D. (1999). Violence risk assessment: Science and practice. *Legal and Criminological Psychology*, *4*, 149-184.

Douglas, K.S., & Webster, C.D. (1999). Predicting violence in mentally and personality disordered individuals. In R. Roesch, S.D. Hart, & J.R.P. Ogloff (Eds.), *Psychology and law: The state of the discipline* (pp. 175-239). New York: Plenum.

Douglas, K.S., Webster, C.D., Hart, S.D., Eaves, D., & Ogloff, J.R. (2001). *HCR-20 Violence Risk Management Companion Guide*. Burnaby, BC, Canada: Mental Health, Law, and Policy Institute, Simon Fraser University.

Eaves, D., Tien, G., & Wilson, D. (2000). Offenders with major affective disorders. In S. Hodgins & R. Müller-Isberner (Eds.), *Violence, crime and mentally disordered offenders* (pp. 131-152). Chichester, UK: Wiley.

Edens, J.F., Buffington-Vollum, J.K., Colwell, K.W., Johnson, D.W., & Johnson, J.K. (2002). Psychopathy and institutional misbehavior among incarcerated sex offenders: A comparison of the Psychopathy Checklist-Revised and the Personality Assessment Inventory. *International Journal of Forensic Mental Health*, *1*, 49-58.

Edens, J.F., Petrila, J., & Buffington-Vollum, J.K. (2001). Psychopathy and the death penalty: Can the Psychopathy Checklist-Revised identify offenders who represent "a continuing threat to society?" *Journal of Psychiatry and the Law*, 29, 433-481.

Edens, J.F., Poythress, N.G., & Lilienfeld, S.O. (1999). Identifying inmates at risk for disciplinary incidents: A comparison of two measures of psychopathy. *Behavioral Sciences and the Law*, *17*, 435-443.

Edens, J.F., Skeem, J.L., Cruise, K.R., & Cauffman, E. (2001). Assessment of "juvenile psychopathy" and its association with violence: A critical review. *Behavioral Sciences and the Law*, *19*, 53-80.

Ekblom, B. (1970). *Acts of violence by patients in mental hospitals*. Uppsala, Sweden: Almqvist & Wiksells.

Emmerik, J.L. van (1985). *TBS en recidive: Een beschrijving van ter beschikking gestelden van wie de maatregel is beëindigd in de periode 1974-1979*. [Recidivism after forensic psychiatric treatment: A description of forensic patients who were released between 1974-1979]. The Hague, the Netherlands: Staatsuitgeverij.

Emmerik, J.L. van (1989). *TBS en recidive: Een beschrijving van ter beschikking gestelden van wie de maatregel is beëindigd in de periode 1979-1983.* [Recidivism after forensic psychiatric treatment: A description of forensic patients who were released between 1973-1983]. Arnhem, the Netherlands: Gouda Quint.

Emmerik, J.L. van, & Brouwers, M. (2001). *De terbeschikkingstelling in maat en getal: Een beschrijving van de tbs-populatie in de periode 1995-2000* [The tbs-order in numbers and figures: A description of the tbs population in the period 1995-2000]. The Hague, the Netherlands: Dienst Justitiële Inrichtingen.

Exner, J.E., Jr. (1993). *The Rorschach: A Comprehensive System* (Vol.1, 3rd ed.). New York: Wiley.

Exner, J.E., Jr. (2001). *A Rorschach workbook for the Comprehensive System.* Ashville, NC: Rorschach Workshops.

Exner, J.E., & Andronikof-Sanglade, A. (1992). Rorschach changes following brief and short-term therapy. *Journal of Personality Assessment, 59,* 59-71.

Exner, J.E., Kinder, B.N., & Curtis, G. (1995). Reviewing basic design features. In J.E. Exner (Ed.), *Issues and methods in Rorschach research* (pp. 145-158). Mahwah, NJ: Erlbaum.

Eysenck, H.J. (1964). *Crime and personality.* London: Routledge and Kegan Paul.

Eysenck, H.J. (1998). Personality and crime. In T. Millon, E. Simonson, M. Birket-Smith, & R.D. Davis (Eds.), *Psychopathy: Antisocial, criminal, and violent behavior* (pp. 40-49). New York: Guilford.

Fisher, L., & Blair, R.J.R. (1998). Cognitive impairment and its relationship to psychopathic tendencies in children with emotional, and behavioral difficulties. *Journal of Abnormal Child Psychology, 103,* 700-707.

Fleiss, J.L. (1981). *Statistical methods for rates and proportions.* New York: Wiley.

Fleiss, J.L. (1986). *The design and analysis of clinical experiments.* New York: Wiley.

Fleiss, J.L, Wiliams, J.B.W., & Dubro, A.F. (1986). The logistic regression analysis of psychiatric data. *Journal of Psychiatric Research, 20,* 145-209.

Flor, H., Birbaumer, N., Hermann, C., Ziegler, S., & Patrick, C.J. (2002). Aversive Pavlovian conditioning in psychopaths: Peripheral and central correlates. *Psychophysiology*, *39*, 505-518.

Floyd, F.J., & Widaman, K.F. (1995). Factor analysis in the development and refinement of clinical assessment instruments. *Psychological Assessment*, *7*, 286-299.

Forth, A.E., Brown, S.L., Hart, S.D., & Hare, R.D. (1996). The assessment of psychopathy in male and female noncriminals: Reliability and validity. *Personality and Individual Differences, 20*, 531-543.

Forth, A.E., & Burke, E. (1998). Psychopathy in adolescence: Assessment, violence, and developmental precursors. In D.J. Cooke, A.E. Forth, & R.D. Hare (Eds.), *Psychopathy: Theory, research, and implications for society* (pp. 205-229). Dordrecht, the Netherlands: Kluwer.

Forth, A.E., Hart, S.D., & Hare, R.D. (1990). Assessment of psychopathy in male young offenders. *Psychological Assessment: A Journal of Consulting and Clinical Psychology*, *2*, 342-344.

Forth, A.E., Kosson, D.S., & Hare, R.D. (in press). *The Hare Psychopathy Checklist: Youth Version*. Toronto, Ontario, Canada: Multi-Health Systems.

Forth, A.E., & Mailloux, D.L. (2000). Psychopathy in youth: What do we know? In C.B. Gacono (Ed.), *The clinical and forensic assessment of psychopathy: A practitioner's guide* (pp. 25-54). Mahwah, NJ: Erlbaum.

Frick, P. (1998). Callous-unemotional traits and conduct problems: Applying the two-factor model of psychopathy to children. In D.J. Cooke, A.E. Forth, & R.D. Hare (Eds.), *Psychopathy: Theory, research, and implications for society* (pp. 161-187). Dordrecht, the Netherlands: Kluwer.

Frick, P.J. (2002). Juvenile psychopathy from a developmental perspective: Implications for construct development and use in forensic assessments. *Law and Human Behavior, 26*, 247-253.

Frick, P.J., & Ellis, M. (1999). Callous-unemotional traits and subtypes of conduct disorder. *Clinical Child and Family Psychology Review*, *2*, 149-168.

Fulero, S.M. (1995). Review of the Hare Psychopathy Checklist-Revised. In J.C. Conoley & J.C. Impara (Eds.), *Twelfth mental measurements yearbook* (pp. 453-454). Lincoln, NE: Buros Institute.

Furby, L., Weinrott, M.R., & Blackshaw, L. (1989). Sex offender recidivism: A review. *Psychological Bulletin, 105*, 303-330.

Furr, K. (1993). Prediction of sexual or violent recidivism among sexual offenders: A comparison of prediction instruments. *Annals of Sex Research, 6*, 271-286.

Gacono, C.B. (1988). *A Rorschach analysis of object relations and defensive structure and their relationship to narcissism and psychopathy in a group of antisocial offenders.* Unpublished doctoral dissertation, United States International University, San Diego.

Gacono, C.B., Meloy, J.R., Sheppard, K., Speth, E., & Roske, A. (1995). A clinical investigation of malingering and psychopathy in hospitalized insanity acquittees. *Bulletin of the American Academy of Psychiatry and Law, 23*, 387-397.

Gendreau, P.P., Goggin, C., & Smith, P. (2002). Is the PCL-R really the "unparalled" measure of offender risk? A lesson in knowledge cumulation. *Criminal Justice and Behavior, 29*, 397-426.

Gendreau, P.P., Little, T., & Goggin, C. (1996). A meta-analysis of the predictors of adult offenders: What works! *Criminology, 34*, 575-607.

Graham, J.R. (2000). *MMPI-2: Assessing personality and psychopathology* (3rd ed.). New York: Oxford University Press.

Grann, M., Långström, N., Tengström, A., & Kullgren, G. (1999). Psychopathy (PCL-R) predicts violent recidivism among criminal offenders with personality disorders in Sweden. *Law and Human Behavior, 23*, 205-217.

Grann, M., Långström, N., Tengström, A., & Stålenheim, E.G. (1998). Reliability of file-based retrospective ratings of psychopathy with the PCL-R. *Journal of Personality Assessment, 70*, 416-426.

Green, S.B., Lissitz, R.W., & Mulaik, S.A. (1977). Limitations of coefficient alpha as an index of unidimensionality. *Educational and Psychological Measurement, 37*, 827-838.

Greeven, P.G.J. (1997). *De intramurale behandeling van forensisch psychiatrische patiënten met een persoonlijkheidsstoornis: een empirisch studie.* [Treatment outcome in personality disordered forensic patients: An empirical study]. Doctoral dissertation University of Utrecht. Deventer, the Netherlands: Gouda Quint.

Gresham, F.M., Lane, K.L., & Lambros, K.M. (2000). Comorbidity of conduct problems and ADHD: Identification of fledging psychopaths. *Journal of Emotional and Behavioral Disorders, 8,* 83-93.

Gretton, H.M., McBride, M., Hare, R.D., O'Shaughnessy, R., & Kumka, G. (2001). Psychopathy and recidivism in adolescent sex offenders. *Criminal Justice and Behavior, 28,* 427-449.

Grisso, T. (1998). *Forensic evaluation of juveniles.* Sarasota, Fl: Professional Resource Press.

Grove, W.M., & Meehl, P.E. (1996). Comparative efficiency of informal (subjective, impressionistic) and formal (mechanical, algorithmic) prediction procedures: The clinical-statistical controversy. *Psychology, Public Policy, and Law, 2,* 293-323.

Gunn, J. (1998). Psychopathy: An elusive concept with moral overtones. In T. Millon, E. Simonsen, M. Birketh-Smith, & R.D. Davis (Eds.), *Psychopathy: Antisocial, criminal, and violent behavior* (pp. 32-39). New York: Guilford.

Haapasalo, J., & Pulkkinen, L. (1992). The Psychopathy Checklist and non-violent offender groups. *Criminal Behaviour and Mental Health, 2,* 315-328.

Hall, G.C.N. (1995). Sexual offender recidivism risk: A meta-analysis of treatment studies. *Journal of Clinical and Consulting Psychology, 63,* 802-809.

Hall, G.C.N., & Hirschman, R. (1991). Toward a theory of sexual aggression: A quadripartite model. *Journal of Clinical and Consulting Psychology, 59,* 662-669.

Hanson, R.K. (1998). What do we know about sexual offender risk assessment? *Psychology, Public Policy, and Law, 4,* 50-72.

Hanson, R.K. (2000). Treatment outcome and evaluation problems (and solutions). In D.R. Laws, S.M. Hudson, & T. Ward (Eds.), *Remaking relapse prevention with sex offenders : A sourcebook* (pp. 485-502). Thousand Oaks, CA: Sage.

Hanson, R.K., & Bussière, M.T. (1996). *Predictors of sexual offender recidivism: A meta-analysis.* [User Report No. 1996-04]. Ottawa, Canada: Department of the Solicitor General.

Hanson, R.K., & Bussière, M.T. (1998). Predicting relapse: A meta-analysis of sexual offender recidivism studies. *Journal of Consulting and Clinical Psychology, 66,* 348-362.

Hanson, R.K., Gordon, A., Harris, A.J.R., Marques, J.K., Murphy, W., Quinsey, V.L., & Seto, M.C. (2002). First report of the collaborative outcome data project on the effectiveness of psychological treatment for sex offenders. *Sexual Abuse: A Journal of Research and Treatment, 14,* 169-194.

Hanson, R.K., & Harris, A.J.R. (2000). Where should we intervene? Dynamic predictors of sexual offense recidivism. *Criminal Justice and Behavior, 27,* 6-35.

Hanson, R.K., Morton, K.E., & Harris, A.J.R. (in press). Sexual offender recidivism risk: What we know and what we need to know. In R. Prentky, E. Janus, M. Seto, & A.W. Burgess (Eds.), *Understanding and managing sexually coercive behavior.* New York: Annals of the New York Academy of Sciences.

Hanson, R.K., & Thornton, D. (1999*). Static-99: Improving actuarial risk assessments for sex offenders* [User Report No. 99-02]. Ottawa, Canada: Department of the Solicitor General.

Hare, R.D. (1970). *Psychopathy: Theory and research.* New York: Wiley.

Hare, R.D. (1978). Electrodermal and cardiovascular correlations of psychopathy. In R.D. Hare & D. Schalling (Eds.), *Psychopathic behavior: Approaches to research* (pp. 107-143). Chichester, UK: Wiley.

Hare, R.D. (1980). A research scale for the assessment of psychopathy in criminal populations. *Personality and Individual Differences, 1,* 111-119.

Hare, R.D. (1985). A comparison of procedures for the assessment of psychopathy. *Journal of Consulting and Clinical Psychology, 53,* 7-16.

Hare, R.D. (1991). *The Hare Psychopathy Checklist-Revised.* Toronto, Ontario, Canada: Multi-Health Systems.

Hare, R.D. (1993). *Without conscience: The disturbing world of the psychopaths among us.* New York: Simon & Schuster.

Hare, R.D. (1996). Psychopathy: A clinical construct whose time has come. *Criminal Justice and Behavior, 23*, 25-54.

Hare, R.D. (1998a). Psychopaths and their nature: Implications for the mental health and criminal justice systems. In T. Millon, E. Simonsen, M. Birket-Smith, & R.D. Davis (Eds.), *Psychopathy: Antisocial, criminal, and violent behavior* (pp. 188-212). New York: Guilford.

Hare, R.D. (1998b). Psychopathy, affect and behavior. In D.J. Cooke, A.E. Forth, & R.D. Hare (Eds.), *Psychopathy: Theory, research, and implications for society* (pp. 105-138). Dordrecht, the Netherlands: Kluwer.

Hare, R.D. (1998c). The Hare PCL-R: Some issues concerning its use and misuse. *Legal and Criminological Psychology, 3*, 99-119.

Hare, R.D., Clark, D., Grann, M., & Thornton, D. (2000). Psychopathy and the predictive validity of the PCL-R: An international perspective. *Behavioral Sciences and the Law, 18*, 623-645.

Hare, R.D., & Craigen, D. (1974). Psychopathy and physiological activity in a mixed-motive game situation. *Psychophysiology, 11*, 197-206.

Hare, R.D., Harpur, T.J., Hakstian, A.R., Forth, A.E., Hart, S.D., & Newman, J.P. (1990). The Revised Psychopathy Checklist: Descriptive statistics, reliability, and factor structure. *Psychological Assessment: A Journal of Consulting and Clinical Psychology, 2*, 338-341.

Hare, R.D., Hart, S.D., & Harpur, T.J. (1991). Psychopathy and the proposed DSM-IV criteria for antisocial personality disorder. *Journal of Abnormal Psychology, 100*, 391-398.

Hare, R.D., & Jutai, J. (1988). Psychopathy and cerebral asymmetry in semantic processing. *Personality and Individual Differences, 9*, 329-337.

Hare, R.D., & McPherson, L.M. (1984). Violent and aggressive behavior by criminal psychopaths. *International Journal of Law and Psychiatry, 7*, 35-50.

Hare, R.D., Williamson, S.E., & Harpur, T.J. (1988). Psychopathy and language. In T.E. Moffitt & S.A. Mednick (Eds.), *Biological contributions to crime causation* (pp. 68-92). Dordrecht, the Netherlands: Nijhoff.

Harpur, T.J., & Hare, R.D. (1994). Assessment of psychopathy as a function of age. *Journal of Abnormal Psychology, 103*, 604-609.

Harpur, T.J., Hare, R.D., & Hakstian R. (1989). Two-factor conceptualization of psychopathy: Construct validity and assessment implications. *Psychological Assessment: A Journal of Consulting and Clinical Psychology, 1*, 6-17.

Harpur, T.J., Hakstian, R., & Hare, R.D. (1988). Factor structure of the Psychopathy Checklist. *Journal of Consulting and Clinical Psychology, 56*, 741-747.

Harris, G.T., & Rice, M.E. (1997). Risk appraisal and management of violent behavior. *Psychiatric Services, 48*, 1168-1176.

Harris, G.T., Rice, M.E., & Cormier, C.A. (1991). Psychopathy and violent recidivism. *Law and Human Behavior, 15*, 625-637.

Harris, G.T., Rice, M.E., & Quinsey, V.L. (1993). Violent recidivism of mentally disordered offenders: The development of a statistical prediction instrument. *Criminal Justice and Behavior, 20*, 315-335.

Harris, G.T., Rice, M.E., & Quinsey, V.L. (1994). Psychopathy as a taxon: Evidence that psychopaths are a discrete class. *Journal of Consulting and Clinical Psychology, 62*, 387-397.

Hart, S.D. (1998). The role of psychopathy in assessing risk for violence: Conceptual and methodological issues. *Legal and Criminological Psychology, 3*, 121-137.

Hart, S.D. (2001). Forensic issues. In W.J. Livesley (Ed.), *Handbook of personality disorders: Theory, research, and treatment* (pp. 555-569). New York: Guilford.

Hart, S.D., Cox, D.N., & Hare, R.D. (1995). *Manual for the Psychopathy Checklist: Screening Version (PCL:SV)*. Toronto, Ontario, Canada: Multi-Health Systems.

Hart, S.D., Forth, A.E., & Hare, R.D. (1991). The MCMI-II and psychopathy. *Journal of Personality Disorders, 5*, 318-327.

Hart, S.D., & Hare, R.D. (1989). Discriminant validity of the Psychopathy Checklist in a forensic psychiatric population. *Psychological Assessment: A Journal of Consulting and Clinical Psychology, 1*, 211-218.

Hart, S.D., & Hare, R.D. (1997). Psychopathy: Assessment and association with criminal conduct. In D.M. Stoff, J. Breiling, & J. Maser (Eds.), *Handbook of antisocial behavior* (pp. 22-35). New York: Wiley.

Hart, S.D., Hare, R.D., & Forth, A.E. (1994). Psychopathy as a risk marker for violence: Development and validation of a screening version of the revised Psychopathy Checklist. In J. Monahan & H.J. Steadman (Eds.), *Violence and mental disorder: Developments in risk assessment* (pp. 81-99). Chicago: University of Chicago Press.

Hart, S.D., Hare, R.D., & Harpur, T.J. (1992). The Psychopathy Checklist: Overview for researchers and clinicians. In J. Rosen & P. McReynolds (Eds.), *Advances in psychological assessment* (pp. 103-130). New York: Plenum.

Hart, S.D., Watt, K.A., & Vincent, G.M. (2002). Commentary on Seagrave and Grisso: Impressions of the state of the art. *Law and Human Behavior, 26*, 241-245.

Heilbrun, K., Hart, S.D., Hare, R.D., Gustafson, D., Nunez, C., & White, A.J. (1998). Inpatient and post discharge aggression in mentally disordered offenders: The role of psychopathy. *Journal of Interpersonal Violence, 13*, 514-527.

Hemphill, J.F., Hare, R.D., & Wong, S. (1998). Psychopathy and recidivism: A review. *Legal and Criminological Psychology, 3*, 139-170.

Hemphill, J.F., & Hart, S.D. (2002). Motivating the unmotivated: Psychopathy, treatment, and change. In M. McMurran (Ed.), *Motivating offenders to change* (pp. 193-219). Chichester, UK: Wiley.

Hemphill, J., Hart, S.D., & Hare, R.D. (1994). Psychopathy and substance use. *Journal of Personality Disorders, 8*, 32-40.

Hemphill, J.F., & Howell, A.J. (2000). Adolescent offenders and stages of change. *Psychological Assessment, 12*, 371-381.

Hemphill, J.F., Templeman, R., Hare, R.D., & Wong, S. (1998). Psychopathy and crime: Recidivism and criminal careers. In D.J. Cooke, A.E. Forth, & R.D. Hare (Eds.), *Psychopathy: Theory, research, and implications for society* (pp. 375-399). Dordrecht, the Netherlands: Kluwer.

Henderson, D.K. (1939). *Psychopathic states*. London: Chapman & Hall.

Herpertz, S.C., & Sass, H. (2000). Emotional deficiency and psychopathy. *Behavioral Sciences and the Law, 18*, 567-580.

Hervé, H.F., & Hare, R.D. (2002). *Criminal psychopathy and its subtypes: Reliability and generalizability.* Paper presented at the 2002 Biennial Conference of the American Psyhology-Law Society (AP-LS), Austin, TX.

Hicks, M.M., Rogers, R., & Cashel, M.L. (2000). Predictions of violent and total incidents among institutionalized male juvenile offenders. *Journal of the American Academy of Psychiatry and Law, 28*, 183-190.

Hildebrand, M., & Ruiter, C. de (1999). Classificatie en diagnostiek bij forensisch psychiatrische patiënten. [Classification and assessment of forensic psychiatric patients]. In C. de Ruiter & M. Hildebrand (Red.), *Behandelingsstrategieën bij forensisch psychiatrische patiënten* (pp. 1-8). Houten, the Netherlands: Bohn Stafleu Van Loghum.

Hildebrand, M., & Ruiter, C. de (2004). PCL-R psychopathy and its relation to DSM-IV Axis I and Axis II disorders in a sample of male forensic psychiatric patients in the Netherlands. *International Journal of Law and Psychiatry, 27*, 233-248.

Hildebrand, M., Ruiter, C. de, & Beek, D.J. van (2001). *SVR-20: Richtlijnen voor het beoordelen van het risico van seksueel gewelddadig gedrag.* [SVR-20: Guidelines for the assessment of risk of sexual violence]. Utrecht, the Netherlands: Forum Educatief.

Hildebrand, M., Ruiter, C. de, & Nijman, H. (2004). PCL-R psychopathy predicts disruptive behavior among male offenders in a Dutch forensic psychiatric hospital. *Journal of Interpersonal Violence, 19*, 13-29.

Hildebrand, M., Ruiter, C. de, & Vogel, V. de (2003). Recidive van verkrachters en aanranders na tbs: De relatie met psychopathie en seksuele deviatie. [Recidivism of rapists after tbs: The relation with psychopathy and sexual deviance]. *De Psycholoog, 38*, 114-124.

Hildebrand, M., Ruiter, C. de, & Vogel, V. de (2004). Psychopathy and sexual deviance in treated rapists: Association with sexual and non-sexual recidivism. *Sexual Abuse: A Journal of Research and Treatment, 16*, 1-24.

Hildebrand, M., Ruiter, C. de, Vogel, V. de, & Wolf, P. van der (2002). Reliability and factor structure of the Dutch language version of Hare's Psychopathy Checklist-Revised. *International Journal of Forensic Mental Health, 1*, 139-154.

Hill, C.D., Rogers, R., & Bickford, M.E. (1996). Predicting aggressive and socially disruptive behavior in a maximum security forensic psychiatric hospital. *Journal of Forensic Sciences, 41,* 56-59.

Hobson, J., & Shine, J. (1998). Measurement of psychopathy in a UK prison population referred for long-term psychotherapy. *British Journal of Criminology, 38,* 504-515.

Hobson, J., Shine, J., & Roberts, R. (2000). How do psychopaths behave in a prison therapeutic community? *Psychology, Crime, and Law, 6,* 139-154.

Hoge, R.D., & Andrews, D.A. (1996). *Assessing the youthful offender: Issues and techniques.* New York: Plenum.

Hoge, R.D., Andrews, D.A., & Leschied, A.W. (1996). An investigation of risk and protective factors in a sample of youthful offenders. *Journal of Child Psychology and Psychiatry, 37,* 419-424.

Holmes, C.A. (1992). Psychopathic disorder: A category mistake. *Journal of Medical Ethics, 17,* 77-85.

Howland, E.W., Kosson, D.S., Patterson, C.M., & Newman, J.P. (1993). Altering a dominant response: Performance of psychopaths and low-socialization college students on a cued reaction time task. *Journal of Abnormal Psychology, 102,* 379-387.

Hughes, G., Hogue, T., Hollin, C., & Champion, H. (1997). First-stage evaluation of a treatment programme for personality disordered offenders. *The Journal of Forensic Psychiatry, 8,* 515-527.

Hunter, M., & Carmel, H. (1992). The cost of staff injuries from inpatient violence. *Hospital and Community Psychiatry, 43,* 586-588.

Intrator, J., Hare, R.D., Stritske, P., Brichtswein, K., Dorfman, D., Harpur, T., Bernstein, D., Handelsman, L., Schaefer, C., Keilp, J., Rosen, J., & Machac, J. (1997). A brain imaging (SPECT) study of semantic and affective processing in psychopaths. *Biological Psychiatry, 42,* 96-103.

Jenkins, R. (1960). The psychopathic or antisocial personality. *Journal of Nervous and Mental Disease, 131,* 318-334.

Jong, C.A.J. de, Brink, W. van den, & Jansma, A. (2000). *ICL-R: Handleiding bij de vernieuwde Nederlandse versie van de Interpersonal Checklist (ICL).* [Manual of the revised Dutch version of the Interpersonal Checklist (ICL)]. Sint Oedenrode, the Netherlands: Novadic.

Jong, C.A.J. de, Derks, F.C.H., Oel, C.J van, & Rinne, Th. (1997). *Gestructureerd Interview voor de DSM-IV Persoonlijkheidsstoornissen* [Structured Interview for DSM-IV Personality Disorders]. Sint Oedenrode, the Netherlands: Stichting Verslavingszorg Oost Brabant.

Johns, J.H., & Quay, H.C. (1962). The effect of social reward on verbal conditioning in psychopathic and neurotic military offenders. *Journal of Consulting Psychology, 26,* 217-220.

Jöreskog, K.G., & Sörbom, D. (1993). *Lisrel 8: Structural equation modeling with the SIMPLIS command language.* Chicago: Scientific Software.

Karpman, B. (1941). On the need for separating psychopathy into two distinct clinical types: Symptomatic and idiopathic. *Journal of Criminology and Psychopathology, 3,* 112-137.

Karpman, B. (1946). A yardstick for measuring psychopathy. *Federal Probation, 10,* 26-31.

Karpman, B. (1948). The myth of the psychopathic personality. *American Journal of Psychiatry, 104,* 523-534.

Karpman, B. (1961). The structure of neurosis: With special differentials between neurosis, psychosis, homosexuality, alcoholism, psychopathy, and criminality. *Archives of Criminal Psychodynamics, 4,* 599-646.

Karson, C., & Bigelow, L.B. (1987). Violent behavior in schizophrenic inpatients. *The Journal of Nervous and Mental Disease, 175,* 161-164.

Kay, S.R., Wolkenfeld, F., & Murrill, L.M. (1988). Profiles of aggression among psychiatric patients II: Covariates and predictors. *Journal of Nervous and Mental Disease, 176,* 547-557.

Kendell, R.E. (1989). Clinical validity. *Psychological Medicine, 19,* 45-55.

Kiehl, K.A., Smith, A.M., Hare, R.D., Mendrek, A., Forster, B.B., Brink, J., & Liddle, P.F. (2001). Limbic abnormalities in affective processing by criminal psychopaths as revealed by functional magnetic resonance imaging. *Biological Psychiatry, 50,* 677-684.

Kline, R.B. (1998). *Principles and practice of structural equation modeling*. New York: Guilford.

Koch, J.L. (1891). *Die psychopathischen Minderwertigkeiten*. Ravensburg, Germany: Maier.

Koivisto, H., & Haapasalo, J. (1996). Childhood malreatment and adulthood psychopathy in light of file-based assessments among mental state examinees. *Studies on Crime and Crime Prevention, 5*, 91-104.

Kosson, D.S., Cyterski, T.D., Steuerwald, B.L., Neumann, C.S., & Walker-Matthews, S. (2002). The reliability and validity of the Psychopathy Checklist: Youth Version (PCL:YV) in nonincarcerated adolescent males. *Psychological Assessment, 14*, 97-109.

Kosson, D.S., Smith, S.S., & Newman, J.P. (1990). Evaluating the construct validity of psychopathy in Black and White male inmates: Three preliminary studies. *Journal of Abnormal Psychology, 3*, 250-259.

Kosson, D.S., Steuerwald, B.L., Forth, A.E., & Kirkhart, K.J. (1997). A new method for assigning the interpersonal behavior of psychopathic individuals: Preliminary validation studies. *Psychological Assessment, 9*, 89-101.

Kraemer, H.C., Kazdin, A.E., Offord, D.R., Kessler, R.C., Jensen, P.S., Kupfer, D.J. (1997). Coming to terms with the terms of risk. *Archives of General Psychiatry, 54*, 337-343.

Kraepelin, E. (1915). *Psychiatrie: Ein Lehrbuch* (8th ed., Vol. 4). Leipzig, Germany: Barth.

Kropp, P.R., Hart, S.D., Webster, C.D., & Eaves, D. (1994*). Manual for the Spousal Assault Risk Assessment Guide*. Vancouver, Canada: British Columbia Institute for Family Violence.

Kroner, D.G., & Mills, J.F. (2001). The accuracy of five risk appraisal instruments in predicting institutional misconduct and new convictions. *Criminal Justice and Behavior, 28*, 471-489.

Kullgren, G., Grann, M., & Holmberg, G. (1996). The Swedish forensic concept of severe mental disorder as related to personality disorders. *International Journal of Law and Psychiatry, 19*, 191-200.

LaForge, R., & Suczek, R.F. (1955). The interpersonal dimension of personality: III. An interpersonal checklist. *Journal of Personality*, *24*, 94-112.

Lapierre, D., Braun, C.M.J., & Hodgins, S. (1995). Ventral frontal deficits in psychopathy: Neuropsychological test findings. *Neuropsychologia*, *11*, 139-151.

Laws, D.R. (1989). *Relapse prevention with sex offenders*. New York: Guilford.

Leuw, E. (1995). *Recidive na ontslag uit de TBS*. [Recidivism after forensic psychiatric treatment]. Arnhem, the Netherlands: Gouda Quint.

Leuw, E. (1999). *Recidive na de TBS: patronen, trends en de inschatting van gevaar*. [Recidivism after forensic psychiatric treatment: Patterns, trends, processes and risk assessment]. Arnhem, the Netherlands: Gouda Quint.

Levenson, M.R., Kiehl, K.A., & Fitzpatrick, C.M. (1995). Assessing psychopathic attributes in a noninstitutionalized population. *Journal of Personality and Social Psychology*, *68*, 151-158.

Lewis, A. (1974). Psychopathic personality: A most elusive category. *Psychological Medicine*, *4*, 133-140.

Lilienfeld, S.O. (1994). Conceptual problems in the assessment of psychopathy. *Clinical Psychology Review*, *14*, 17-38.

Lilienfeld, S.O., Purcell, C., & Jones-Alexander, J. (1997). Assessment of antisocial behavior in adults. In D.M. Stoff, J. Breiling, & J. Maser (Eds.), *Handbook of antisocial behavior* (pp. 60-74). New York: Wiley.

Linehan, M.M. (1993). *Cognitive-behavioral treatment of borderline personality disorder*. New York: Guilford.

Lion, J.R., & Reid, W.H. (Eds.) (1983). *Assaults within psychiatric facilities*. New York: Grune and Stratton.

Litwack, T.R. (2001). Actuarial versus clinical assessments of dangerousness. *Psychology, Policy, and Law*, *7*, 409-443.

Litwack, T.R., & Schlesinger, L.B. (1987). Assessing and predicting violence: Research, law and implications. In A. Hess & I. Weiner (Eds.), *Handbook of forensic psychology* (pp. 205-257). New York: Wiley.

Livesley, W.J. (1998). Suggestions for a framework for an empirically based classification of personality disorder. *Canadian Journal of Psychiatry*, *43*, 137-147.

Logan, C., Blackburn, R., Donnelly, J., & Renwick, S. (2002, March). *Personality disorders, psychopathy and other mental disorders: Co-morbidity among patients at English and Scottish high security hospitals*. Paper presented at the Second Annual Congress of the International Association of Forensic Mental Health Services, Munich, Germany.

Looman, J., Abracen, J., & Nicholaichuck, T.P. (2000). Recidivism among treated sexual offenders and matched controls: Data from the Regional Treatment Centre (Ontario). *Journal of Interpersonal Violence, 15*, 279-290.

Looman, J., Abracen, J., Serin, R., & Marquis, P. (2002). *Psychopathy, treatment change and recidivism in high risk need sexual offenders*. Manuscript submitted for publication.

Loranger, A.W. (1992). Are current self-report and interview measures adequate for epidemiological studies of personality disorders? *Journal of Personality Disorders, 6*, 313-325.

Lösel, F. (1998). Treatment and management of psychopaths. In D.J. Cooke, A.E. Forth, & R.D. Hare (Eds.), *Psychopathy: Theory, research, and implications for society* (pp. 303-354). Dordrecht, the Netherlands: Kluwer.

Lykken, D.T. (1995). *The antisocial personalities*. Hillsdale, NJ: Erlbaum.

Lynam, D.R. (2002). Fledging psychopathy: A view from personality theory. *Law and Human Behavior, 26*, 255-259.

Lyon, D.R., & Ogloff, J.R.P. (2000). Legal and ethical issues in psychopathy assessment. In C.B. Gacono (Ed.), *The clinical and forensic assessment of psychopathy: A practitioner's guide* (pp. 139-173). Mahwah, NJ: Erlbaum.

Mailloux, D.L., Forth, A.E., & Kroner, D.G. (1997). Psychopathy and substance use in adolescent male offenders. *Psychological Reports, 80*, 529-530.

Maletzky, B.M. (1996). Denial of treatment or treatment of denial? *Sexual Abuse: A Journal of Research and Treatment, 8*, 1-15.

Malsch, M., & Hielkema, J. (1999). Forensic assessment in Dutch criminal insanity cases: Participants' perspectives. In M. Malsch & J.F. Nijboer (Eds.), *Complex cases: Perspectives on the Netherlands criminal justice system* (pp. 213-228). Amsterdam: Thela Thesis.

Mann, R.E. (2000). Managing resistance and rebellion in relapse prevention intervention. In D.R. Laws, S.M. Hudson, & T. Ward (Eds.), *Remaking relapse prevention with sex offenders: A sourcebook* (pp. 187-200). Thousand Oaks, CA: Sage.

Mann, R.E., & Rollnick, S.(1996). Motivational interviewing with a sex offender who believed he was innocent. *Behavioural and Cognitive Psychotherapy, 24*, 127-134.

Marle, H.J.C. van (2002). The Dutch Entrustment Act (TBS): Its principles and innovations. *International Journal of Forensic Mental Health, 1*, 83-92.

Marques, J.K. (1999). How to answer the question "does sex offender treatment work?" *Journal of Interpersonal Violence, 14*, 437-451.

Marshall, W.L. (1994). Treatment effects on denial and minimization in incarcerated sex offenders. *Behaviour Research and Therapy, 32*, 559-564.

Marx, B.P., Miranda, R., & Meyerson, L.A. (1999). Cognitive-behavioral treatment for rapists: Can we do better? *Clinical Psychology Review, 19*, 875-894.

Maudsley, H. (1874). *Responsibility in mental diseases*. London: King.

McConnaughy, E.A. (1987). The person of the therapist in psychotherapeutic practice. *Psychotherapy, 24*, 303-314.

McCord, W., & McCord, J. (1964). *The psychopath: An essay on the criminal mind*. Princeton, NJ: Van Nostrand.

McDermott, P.A., Alterman, A.I., Cacciola, J.S., Rutherford, M.J., Newman, J.P., & Mulholland, J.P. (2000). Generality of Psychopathy Checklist-Revised factors over prisoners and substance-dependent patients. *Journal of Consulting and Clinical Psychology, 68*, 181-186.

McGraw, K.O., & Wong, S.P. (1996). Forming inferences about some intraclass correlation coefficients. *Psychological Methods, 1*, 30-46.

McInerny, T. (2000). Dutch TBS forensic services: A personal view. *Criminal Behaviour and Mental Health, 10*, 213-228.

Meehl, P.E. (1995). Bootstrap taxometrics: Solving the classification problem in psychopathology. *American Psychologist, 50*, 266-275.

Megargee, E.I. (1976). The prediction of dangerous behavior. *Criminal Justice and Behavior, 3*, 3-21.

Megargee, E.I., & Bohn, M.J., Jr. (1979). *Classifying criminal offenders. A new system based on the MMPI.* Beverly Hills, CA: Sage.

Megargee, E.I., Cook, P.E., & Mendelsohn, G.E. (1967). Development and validation of an MMPI scale of assaultiveness in overcontrolled individuals. *Journal of Abnormal Psychology, 72,* 519-528.

Meloy, J.R. (1988). *The psychopathic mind: Origins, dynamics, and treatment.* Northvale, NJ: Aronson.

Meloy, J.R, & Gacono, C. (1995). Assessing the psychopathic personality. In J.N. Butcher (Ed.), *Clinical personality assessment: Practical approaches* (pp. 410-422). New York: Oxford University Press.

Melton, G.B., Petrila, J., Poythress, N.G., & Slobogin, C. (1997). *Psychological evaluations for the courts: A handbook for mental health professionals and lawyers* (2nd ed.). New York: Guilford.

Menzies, R., & Webster, C.D. (1995). Construction and validation of risk assessments in a six year follow-up of forensic patients: A tridimensional analysis. *Journal of Consulting and Clinical Psychology, 63,* 766-778.

Meyer, G.J. (1997). On the integration of personality assessment method: The Rorschach and MMPI. *Journal of Personality Assessment, 68,* 297-330.

Meyer, G.J., Finn, S.E., Eyde, L.D., Kay, G.G., Moreland, K.L., Dies, R.R., Eisman, E.J., Kubiszyn, T.W., & Reed, G.M. (2000). Psychological testing and psychological assessment: A review of evidence and issues. *American Psychologist, 56,* 128-165.

Meyers, W.C., Burkett, R.C., & Harris, H.E. (1995). Adolescent psychopathy in relation to delinquent behaviors, conduct disorder, and personality disorders. *Journal of Forensic Sciences, 40,* 435-439.

Miller, W.R., & Rollnick, S. (Eds.) (1991). *Motivational Interviewing: Preparing people to change addictive behavior.* New York: Guilford.

Miller, W.R., & Tonigan, J.S. (1996). Assessing drinkers' motivation for change: The stages of changes readiness and treatment eagerness scale (SOCRATES). *Psychology of Addictive Behaviors, 10,* 81-89.

Millon, T. (1969). *Modern psychopathology: A biosocial approach to maladaptive learning functioning.* Philadelphia: Saunders.

Millon, T. (1981). *Disorders of personality: DSM-III: Axis II.* New York: Wiley.

Millon, T., & Davis, R.D. (1998). Ten subtypes of psychopathy. In T. Millon, E. Simonson, M. Birket-Smith, & R.D. Davis (Eds.), *Psychopathy: Antisocial, criminal, and violent behavior* (pp. 161-170). New York: Guilford.

Millon, T., Simonsen, E., & Birket-Smith, M. (1998). Historical conceptions of psychopathy in the United States and Europe. In T. Millon, E. Simonson, M. Birket-Smith, & R.D. Davis (Eds.), *Psychopathy: Antisocial, criminal, and violent behavior* (pp. 3-31). New York: Guilford.

Moffitt, T.E. (1993). Adolescence-limited and life-course persistent antisocial behavior: A developmental approach. *Psychological Review, 100,* 674-701.

Moltó, J., Poy, R., & Torrubia, R. (2000). Standardization of the Hare Psychopathy Checklist-Revised in a Spanish prison sample. *Journal of Personality Disorders, 14,* 84-96.

Monahan, J. (1981). *Predicting violent behavior: An assessment of clinical techniques.* Beverly Hills, CA: Sage.

Monahan, J., & Appelbaum, P.S. (2000). Reducing violence risk: Diagnostically based clues from the McArthur Violence Risk Assessment Study. In S. Hodgins (Ed.), *Violence among the mentally ill: Effective treatments and management strategies* (pp. 19-34). Boston: Kluwer.

Monahan, J., & Steadman, H.J. (Eds.) (1994). *Violence and mental disorder: Developments in risk assessment.* Chicago: University of Chicago Press.

Monahan, J., & Steadman, H.J., Silver, E., Appelbaum, P.S., Robbins, P.C., Mulvey, E.P., Roth, L.H., Grisso, T., & Banks, S. (2001). *Rethinking risk assessment: The MacArthur study of mental disorder and violence.* New York: Oxford University Press.

Mossman, D. (1994). Assessing predictions of violence: Being accurate about accuracy. *Journal of Consulting and Clinical Psychology, 62,* 783-792.

Motiuk, L.L. (1995). Refocusing the role of psychology in risk assessment: Assessment, communication, monitoring, and intervention. In T.A. Leis, L.L. Motiuk, & J.R. Ogloff (Eds.), *Forensic psychology: Policy and practice in corrections.* Canada: Correctional Service of Canada.

Müller-Isberner, R. (1993). Managing insane offenders. *International Bulletin of Law & Mental Health, 4*, 28-30.

Myers, W.C., Burket, R.C., & Harris, E.H. (1995). Adolescent psychopathy in relation to delinquent behaviors, conduct disorder, and personality disorders. *Journal of Forensic Sciences, 40*, 436-440.

Nedopil, N., Hollweg, M., Hartmann, J., & Jasper, R. (1998). Comorbidity of psychopathy with major mental disorders. In D.J. Cooke, A.E. Forth, & R.D. Hare (Eds.), *Psychopathy: Theory, research and implications for society* (pp. 257-268). Dordrecht, the Netherlands: Kluwer.

Newman, J.P. (1998). Psychopathic behavior: An information processing perspective. In D.J. Cooke, A.E. Forth, & R.D. Hare (Eds.), *Psychopathy: Theory, research and implications for society* (pp. 81-104). Dordrecht, the Netherlands: Kluwer.

Newman, J.P., Kosson, D.S., & Paterson, C.M. (1992). Delay of gratification in psychopathic and nonpsychopathic offenders. *Journal of Abnormal Psychology, 101*, 630-636.

Newman, J.P., & Wallace, J.F. (1993). Psychopathy and cognition. In P.C. Kendall & K.S. Dobson (Eds.), *Psychopathy and cognition* (pp. 293-349). New York: Academic Press.

Niemantsverdriet, J.R. (1993). *Achteraf bezien: over het evalueren van ter beschikking stellingen.* [In retrospect: Evaluating committals to a forensic mental hospital]. Doctoral dissertation University of Nijmegen. Utrecht, the Netherlands: Elinkwijk.

Novaco, R.W. (1994). Anger as a risk factor for violence among the mentally disordered. In J. Monahan & H. Steadman (Eds.), *Violence and mental disorder: Developments in risk assessment* (pp. 21-59). Chicago: University of Chicago Press.

Nijman, H.L.I. (1999). *Aggressive behavior of psychiatric inpatients: Measurement, prevalence, and determinants.* Doctoral dissertation University Maastricht. Maastricht, the Netherlands: Datawyse/Universitaire Pers Maastricht.

Nijman, H.L.I., Allertz, W.W.F., Merckelbach, H.L.G.J., Campo, J. à, & Ravelli, D. (1997). Aggressive behaviour on an acute psychiatric admissions ward. *European Journal of Psychiatry, 11*, 106-114.

O'Brien, B.S., & Frick, P.J. (1996). Reward dominance: Associations with anxiety, conduct problems, and psychopathy in children. *Journal of Abnormal Child Psychology, 24*, 223-240.

Ogloff, J.R.P., & Lyon, D.R. (1998). Legal issues associated with the concept of psychopathy. In D.J. Cooke, A.E. Forth, & R.D. Hare (Eds.), *Psychopathy: Theory, research and implications for society* (pp. 401-422). Dordrecht, the Netherlands: Kluwer.

Ogloff, J., Wong, S., & Greenwood, A. (1990). Treating criminal psychopaths in a therapeutic community program. *Behavioral Sciences and the Law, 8*, 81-90.

O'Kane, A., Fawcett, D., & Blackburn, R. (1996). Psychopathy and moral reasoning: A comparison of two classifications. *Personality and Individual Differences, 20*, 505-514.

O'Neill, M.L., Lidz, V., & Heilbrun, K. (2003). Adolescents with psychopathic characteristics in a substance abusing cohort: Treatment process and outcomes. *Law and Human Behavior, 27*, 299-313.

Partridge, G. (1930). Current conceptualizations of psychopathic personality. *American Journal of Psychiatry, 10*, 53-99.

Patrick, C.J. (1994). Emotion and psychopathy: Startling new insights. *Psychophysiology, 31*, 319-330.

Patrick, C.J., Bradley, M.M., & Lang, P.J. (1993). Emotion in the criminal psychopath: Startle reflex modulation. *Journal of Abnormal Psychology, 102*, 82-92.

Patrick, C.J., Cuthbert, B.N., & Lang, P.J. (1994). Emotion in the criminal psychopath: Fear imaging processing. *Journal of Abnormal Psychology, 103*, 523-534.

Pfohl, B., Blum, N., & Zimmerman, M. (1995*). Structured Interview for DSM-IV Personality* (DSM-IV). Iowa City, IA: Department of Psychiatry, University of Iowa.

Pfohl, B., Blum, N., & Zimmerman, M., & Stangl, D. (1989). *Structured Interview for DSM-III-R Personality* (SIDP-R). Iowa City, IA: Department of Psychiatry, University of Iowa.

Pham, T., Remy, S., Dailliet, A., & Lienard, L. (1998). Psychopathie et évolution des comportements violents en milieu psychiatrique de sécurité. *L'Encéphale*, *24*, 173-179.

Pinel, P. (1962). *A treatise on insanity* (D. Davis, Trans.). New York: Hafner. (Original work published 1801)

Plutchik, R. (1995). Outward and inward directed aggressiveness: The interaction between violence and suicidality. *Pharmacopsychiatry*, *28*, 47-57.

Porter, S. (1996). Without conscience or without active conscience? The etiology of psychopathy revisited. *Aggression and Violent Behavior*, *1*, 179-189.

Porter, S., Fairweather, D., Drugge, J., Hervé, H., Birt, A., & Boer, D.P. (2000). *Criminal Justice and Behavior*, *27*, 216-233.

Prentky, R.A., Lee, A.F.S., Knight, R.A., & Cerce, D.D. (1997). Recidivism rates among child molesters and rapists: A methodological analysis. *Law and Human Behavior*, *6*, 635-659.

Prichard, J.C (1835). *A treatise on insanity and other disorders affecting the mind.* London: Sherwood, Gilbert, & Piper.

Prochaska, J.O., & DiClemente, C.C. (1986). Toward a comprehensive model of change. In W. R. Miller & N. Heather (Eds.), *Addictive Behaviors: Processes of change* (pp. 3-27). New York: Plenum.

Prochaska, J.O., DiClemente, C.C., & Norcross, J.C. (1992). In search of how people change: Applications to addictive behaviors. *American Psychologist*, *47*, 1102-1104.

Proulx, J., Pellerin, B., Paradis, Y., McKibben, A., Aubut, J., & Ouimet, M. (1997). Static and dynamic predictors of recidivism in sexual aggressors. *Sexual Abuse: A Journal of Research and Treatment*, *9*, 7-27.

Quay, H.C. (1977). Measuring dimensions of deviant behavior: The Behavior Problem Checklist. *Journal of Abnormal Child Psychology*, *5*, 277-287.

Quinsey, V.L., Harris, G.T., Rice, M.T., & Cormier, C.A. (1998). *Violent offenders: Appraising and managing risk.* Washington, DC: American Psychological Association.

Quinsey, V.L., Lalumière, M.L., Rice, M.E., & Harris, G.T. (1995). Predicting sexual offenses. In J.D. Campbell (Ed.), *Assessing dangerousness: Violence by sexual offenders, batterers, and child abusers* (pp. 114-137). Thousands Oaks, CA: Sage.

Quinsey, V.L., Rice, M.E., & Harris, G.T. (1995). Actuarial prediction of sexual recidivism. *Journal of Interpersonal Violence, 10*, 85-115.

Raine, A. (1985). A psychometric assessment of Hare's checklist for psychopathy on an English prison population. *British Journal of Clinical Psychology, 24*, 247-258.

Raine, A. (2001). Psychopathy, violence, and brain imaging. In A. Raine & J. Sanmartin (Eds.), *Violence and psychopathy* (pp. 35-56). New York: Academic Press.

Raine, A., Lencz, T., T., Bihrle, S., LaCasse, L., & Colletti, P. (2000). Reduced prefrontal gray matter volume and reduced autonomic activity in antisocial personality disorder. *Archives of General Psychiatry, 57*, 119-127.

Raine, A. & Venables, P.H. (1988a). Skin conductance responsivity in psychopaths to orienting, defensive, and consonant-vowel stimuli. *Journal of Psychophysiology, 2*, 221-225.

Raine, A., & Venables, P.H. (1988b). Enhanced P3 evoked potentials and longer recovery times in psychopaths. *Psychophysiology, 25*, 30-38.

Rasmussen, K., & Levander, S. (1996). Individual rather than situational characteristics predict violence in a maximum security hospital. *Journal of Interpersonal Violence, 11*, 376-390.

Rasmussen K, Storsæter, O., & Levander S. (1999). Personality disorders, psychopathy, and crime in a Norwegian prison population. *International Journal of Law and Psychiatry, 22*, 91-97.

Reise, S.P., & Oliver, C.J. (1994). Development of a California Q-Set indicator of primary psychopathy. *Journal of Personality Assessment, 62*, 130-144.

Reiss, D., Grubin, D., & Meux, C. (1999). Institutional performance of male 'psychopaths' in a high-security hospital. *Journal of Forensic Psychiatry, 10*, 290-299.

Rice, M.F. (1997). Violent offender research and implications for the criminal justice system. *American Psychologist, 52*, 414-423.

Rice, M.E., & Harris, G.T. (1995a). Violent recidivism: Assessing predictive validity. *Journal of Consulting and Clinical Psychology, 63*, 737-748.

Rice, M.E., & Harris, G.T. (1995b). Psychopathy, schizophrenia, alcohol abuse, and violent recidivism. *International Journal of Law and Psychiatry, 18*, 333-342.

Rice, M.E., & Harris, G.T. (1997a). The treatment of adult offenders. In D.M. Stoff, J. Breiling, & J.D. Maser (Eds.), *Handbook of antisocial behavior* (pp. 425-435). New York: Wiley.

Rice, M.E., & Harris, G.T. (1997b). Cross validation and extension of the Violence Risk Appraisal Guide for child molesters and rapists. *Law and Human Behavior, 21,* 231-241.

Rice, M.E., Harris, G.T., & Cormier, C.A. (1992). An evaluation of a maximum security therapeutic community for psychopaths and other mentally disordered offenders. *Law and Human Behavior, 16,* 399-412.

Rice, M.E., Harris, G.T., & Quinsey, V.L. (1990). A follow-up of rapists assessed in a maximum security psychiatric facility. *Journal of Interpersonal Violence, 5,* 435-448.

Rice, M.E., Harris, G.T., Quinsey, V.L., & Cyr, M. (1990). Planning treatment programs in secure psychiatric facilities. In D.N. Weisstub (Ed.), *Law and mental health: International perspectives* (Vol. 5, pp. 162-230). New York: Pergamon Press.

Robins, L. (1966). *Deviant children grown up: A sociological and psychiatric study of sociopathic personality.* Baltimore: Williams & Wilkins.

Robins, E., & Guze, S.B. (1970). Establishment of diagnostic validity in psychiatric illness: Its application to schizophrenia. *American Journal of Psychiatry, 126,* 983-987.

Rogers, R., Johansen, J., Chang, J.J., & Salekin, R.T. (1997). Predictors of adolescent psychopathy: Oppositional and conduct-disordered symptoms. *Journal of the American Academy of Psychiatry and the Law, 25,* 261-271.

Rogers, R., Salekin, R.T., Hill, C., Sewell, K.W., Murdock, M.E., & Neumann, C.S. (2000). The Psychopathy Checklist-Screening Version: An examination of criteria and subcriteria in three forensic samples. *Assessment, 7,* 1-15.

Rorschach, H. (1942). *Psychodiagnostics: A diagnostic test based on perception.* Bern, Switzerland: Hans Huber. (Original work published 1921)

Rosenbaum, R.L., & Horowitz, M.J. (1983). Motivation for psychotherapy: A factorial and conceptual analysis. *Psychotherapy: Theory, Research, and Practice, 20*, 346-354.

Ross, D.J., Hart, S.D., & Webster, C.D. (1998). *Aggression in psychiatric patients: Using the HCR-20 to assess risk for violence in hospital and in the community.* Vancouver, Canada: Riverview Hospital.

Ruiter, C. de (2003). Diagnostiek en behandeling in de forensische psychiatrie: een pleidooi voor meer evidence-based practice. [Assessment and treatment i Dutch forensic psychiatry: A plea for more evidence-based practice]. In A.H. Schene, Th. Heeren, F. Boer, H. Henselmans, J. van Weeghel, & B. Sabbe (Red.), *Jaarboek Psychiatrie en Psychotherapie* (pp. 187-202). Houten, the Netherlands: Bohn Stafleu Van Loghum.

Ruiter, C. de, & Greeven, P.G.J. (2000). Personality disorders in a Dutch forensic psychiatric sample: Convergence of interview and self-report measures. *Journal of Personality Disorders, 14*, 162-170.

Ruiter, C. de, & Hildebrand, M. Over toerekeningsvatbaarheid. [About criminal responsibility]. In P.J. van Koppen, D.J. Hessing, H.L.G.J. Merkelbach, & H.F.M. Crombag (Eds.), *Het recht van binnen: Psychologie van het recht* (pp. 687-697). Deventer, the Netherlands: Kluwer.

Ruiter, C. de, & Hildebrand, M. (2003). The dual nature of forensic psychiatric practice: Risk assessment and management under the Dutch TBS-order. In P.J. van Koppen & S.D. Penrod (Eds.), *Adversarial versus inquisitorial justice: Psychological perspectives on criminal justice systems* (pp. 91-106). New York: Kluwer/Plenum.

Rush, B. (1812*)*. *Medical inquiries and observations upon diseases of the mind.* Philadelphia: Kimber & Richardson.

Rutherford, M.J., Alterman, A.I., & Cacciola, J.S. (2000). Psychopathy and substance abuse: A bad mix. In C.B. Gacono (Ed.), *The clinical and forensic assessment of psychopathy: A practitioner's guide* (pp. 351-368). Mahwah, NJ: Erlbaum.

Rutherford, M.J., Alterman, A.I., Cacciola, J.S., & McKay, J.R. (1997). Validity of the Psychopathy Checklist-Revised in male methadone patients. *Drug and Alcohol Dependence, 44*, 143-149.

Rutherford, M.J., Cacciola, J.S., Alterman, A.I., & McKay, J.R. (1996). Reliability and validity of the Revised Psychopathy Checklist in women methadone patients. *Assessment, 3*, 43-54.

Rutherford, M.J., Alterman, A.I., Cacciola, J.S., McKay, J.R., & Cook, T.G. (1999). The two-year test-retest reliability of the PCL-R in methadone patients. *Assessment, 6*, 285-291.

Salekin, R.T. (2002). Psychopathy and therapeutic pessimism: Clinical lore or clinical reality? *Clinical Psychology Review, 22*, 79-112.

Salekin, R.T., Rogers, R., & Sewell, K.W. (1996). A review and meta-analysis of the Psychopathy Checklist and Psychopathy Checklist-Revised: Predictive validity of dangerousness. *Clinical Psychology: Science and Practice, 3*, 203-215.

Salekin, R.T., Rogers, R., & Sewell, K.W. (1997). Construct validity of psychopathy in a female offender sample: A multitrait-multimethod evaluation. *Journal of Abnormal Psychology, 106*, 576-585.

Salekin, R.T., Rogers, R., Ustad, K., & Sewell, K.W. (1998). Psychopathy and recidivism among female inmates. *Law and Human Behavior, 22*, 109-128.

Schill, T., & Wang, S. (1990). Correlates of the MMPI-2 anger content. *Psychological Reports, 67*, 800-802.

Schmitt, W.A., & Newman, J.P. (1999). Are all psychopathic individuals low-anxious? *Journal of Abnormal Psychology, 108*, 353-358.

Schneider, K. (1923). *Die psychopathischen Persönlichkeiten.* [The psychopathic personalities]. Vienna: Deuticke.

Schroeder, M.L., Schroeder, K.G., & Hare, R.D. (1983). Generalizability of a checklist for the assessment of psychopathy. *Journal of Consulting and Clinical Psychology, 51*, 511-516.

Seagrave, D., & Grisso, T. (2002). Adolescent development and measurement of juvenile psychopathy. *Law and Human Behavior, 26*, 219-239.

Serin, R.C. (1991). Psychopathy and violence in criminals. *Journal of Interpersonal Violence, 6*, 423-431.

Serin, R.C. (1996). Violent recidivism in criminal psychopaths. *Law and Human Behavior, 20*, 207-217.

Serin, R.C., & Amos, N.L. (1991). The role of psychopathy in the assessment of dangerousness. *International Journal of Law and Psychiatry, 18*, 231-238.

Serin, R.C., & Brown, S.L. (2000). The clinical use of the Hare Psychopathy Checklist-Revised in contemporary risk assessment. In C.B. Gacono (Ed.), *The clinical and forensic assessment of psychopathy: A practitioner's guide* (pp. 251-268). Mahwah, NJ: Erlbaum.

Serin, R.C., & Kennedy, S. (1997). *Treatment readiness and responsivity: Contributing to effective correctional programming.* Research Report R-54. Ottawa, Canada: Correctional Service of Canada.

Serin, R.C., & Kuriychuk, M. (1994). Social and cognitive processing deficits in violent offenders: Implications for treatment. *International Journal of Law and Psychiatry, 17*, 431-441.

Serin, R.C., Mailloux, D.L., & Malcolm, P.B. (2001). Psychopathy, sexual arousal, and recidivism. *Journal of Interpersonal Violence, 16*, 234-246.

Serin, R.C., Malcolm, P.B., Khanna, A., & Barbaree, H.E. (1994). Psychopathy and deviant sexual arousal in incarcerated sexual offenders. *Journal of Interpersonal Violence, 9*, 3-11.

Serin, R.C., Peters, R.D., & Barbaree, H.E. (1990). Predictors of psychopathy and release outcome in a criminal population. *Psychological Assessment: A Journal of Consulting and Clinical Psychology, 2*, 419-422.

Seto, M.C., & Barbaree, H.E. (1999). Psychopathy, treatment behavior, and sex offender recidivism. *Journal of Interpersonal Violence, 14*, 1235-1248.

Seto, M.C., & Lalumière, M.L. (2000). Psychopathy and sexual aggression. In C.B. Gacono (Ed.), *The clinical and forensic assessment of psychopathy: A practitioner's guide* (pp. 333-351). Mahwah, NJ: Erlbaum.

Shah, A., Fineberg, N., & James, D. (1991). Violence among psychiatric inpatients. *Acta Psychiatrica Scandinavica, 84*, 305-309.

Shrout, P.E., & Fleiss, J.L. (1979). Intraclass correlation: Uses in assessing rater reliability. *Psychological Bulletin, 86*, 420-428.

Shrout, P.E., Spitzer, R.L., & Fleiss, J.L. (1987). Quantifications in psychiatric diagnosis revisited. *Archives of General Psychiatry, 44*, 172-177.

Silverthorn, P., & Frick, P.J. (1997). Developmental pathways to antisocial behavior: The delayed-onset pathways in girls. *Development and Psychopathology*, *11*, 101-126.

Simourd, D.J., & Hoge, R.D. (2000). Criminal psychopathy: A risk-and-need perspective. *Criminal Justice and Behavior*, *27*, 256-272.

Sjöstedt, G., & Långström, N. (2002). Assessment of risk for criminal recidivism among rapists: A comparison of four different measures. *Psychology, Crime & Law*, *8*, 25-40.

Skeem, J., & Mulvey, E. (2001). Psychopathy and community violence among civil psychiatric patients: Results from the MacArthur Violence Risk Assessment Study. *Journal of Clinical and Consulting Psychology*, *69*, 358-374.

Skeem, J.L., Mulvey, E.P., & Grisso, T. (2003). Applicability of traditional and revised models of psychopathy to the Psyhopathy Cheklist: Screening Version. *Psychological Assessment*, *15*, 41-55.

Smith, A.M., Gacono, C.B., & Kaufman, L. (1997). A Rorschach comparison of pychopathic and nonpsychopathic conduct disordered adolescents. *Journal of Clinical Psychology*, *53*, 289-300.

Skilling, T.A., Harris, G.T., Rice, M.E., & Quinsey, V.L. (2002). Identifying persistently antisocial offenders using the Hare Psychopathy Checklist and *DSM* antisocial personality disorder criteria. *Psychological Assessment*, *14*, 27-38.

Sloore, H., Derksen, J.J.L., Hellenbosch, G., & Mey, H.R.A. de (1993). *Dutch edition of the Minnesota Multiphasic Personality Inventory-2*. Nijmegen, the Netherlands: PEN.

Smid, W. (2003). *Changes in Rorschach variables of forensic psychiatric patients in residential treatment*. Unpublished master's thesis, University of Amsterdam, the Netherlands.

Smith, S.S., Arnett, P.A., & Newman, J.P. (1992). Neuropsychological differentiation of psychopathic and nonpsychopathic criminal offenders. *Personality and Individual Differences*, *13*, 1233-1243.

Smith, S.S., & Newman, J.P. (1990). Alcohol and drug abuse/dependence disorders in psychopathic and nonpsychopathic criminal offenders. *Journal of Abnormal Psychology*, *99*, 430-439.

Stålenheim, E.G., & Knorring, L. von (1996). Psychopathy and Axis I and Axis II psychiatric disorders in a forensic psychiatric population in Sweden. *Acta Psychiatrica Scandinavica, 94*, 217-223.

Steadman, H., Monahan, J., Appelbaum, P.S., Robbins, P.M., Mulvey, E.P., Grisso, T., Roth, L.H., & Banks, S. (2000). A classification tree approach to the development of actuarial violence risk assessment tools. *Law and Human Behavior, 24*, 83-100.

Stevens, J. (1986). *Applied multivariate statistics for the social sciences*. Hillsdale, NJ: Erlbaum.

Steward, L., & Millson, W.A. (1995). Offender motivation for treatment as a responsivity factor. *Forum on Corrections Research, 7*, 5-7.

Stone, G.L. (1995). Review of the Hare Psychopathy Checklist-Revised. In J.C. Conoley & J.C. Impara (Eds.), *Twelfth mental measurements yearbook* (pp. 454-455). Lincoln, NE: Buros Institute.

Strachan, K., Williamson, S., & Hare, R.D. (1990). *Psychopathy and female offenders*. Unpublished manuscript, Department of psychology, University of British Columbia, Vancouver, Canada.

Streiner, D.L. (1994). Figuring out factors: The use and misuse of factor analysis. *Canadian Journal of Psychiatry, 39*, 135-140.

Tabachnick, B.G., & Fidell, L.S. (2001). *Using multivariate statistics* (4th ed.). Boston: Allyn and Bacon.

Tardiff, K. (1997). Evaluation and treatment of violence patients. In D.M. Stoff, J. Breiling, & J.D. Maser (Eds.), *Handbook of antisocial behavior* (pp. 445-453). New York: Wiley.

Templeman, T.L., & Wollersheim, J.P. (1979). A cognitive-behavioral approach to the treatment of psychopathy. *Psychotherapy: Theory and Research, 16*, 132-139.

Templeman, R., & Wong, S. (1984). Determining the factor structure of the Psychopathy Checklist: A converging approach. *Multivariate Experimental Clinical Research, 10*, 157-166.

Tengström, A., Grann, M., Långström, N., & Kullgren, G. (2000). Psychopathy (PCL-R) as a predictor of violent recidivism among criminal offenders with schizophrenia. *Law and Human Behavior, 24*, 45-58.

Tennent, G., Tennent, D., Prins, H., & Bedford, A. (1990). Psychopathic disorder: A useful concept? *Medicine, Science, and the Law, 30*, 38-44.

Timmerman, I.G.T., & Emmelkamp, P.M.G. (2001). The prevalence and comorbidity of Axis I and Axis II pathology in a group of forensic patients. *International Journal of Offender Therapy and Comparative Criminology, 45*, 198-213.

Toupin, J., Mercier, H., Déry, M., Côté, G., & Hodgins, S. (1995). Validity of the PCL-R for adolescents. *Issues in Criminological and Legal Psychology, 24*, 143-145.

Vertommen, H., Verheul, R., Ruiter, C., de, & Hildebrand, M. (2002). *Handleiding bij de herziene versie van Hare's Psychopathie Checklist*. [Manual of the Dutch version of the revised version of Hare's Psychopathy Checklist]. Lisse, the Netherlands: Swets Test Publishers.

Vogel, V. de, Ruiter, C. de, & Bouman, Y. (2003, July). *Risk assessment and beyond: The construction of checklist of protective factors for (sexually) violent behavior*. Paper presented at the joint conference of the American Psychology-Law Society and the European Association of Psychology and Law. Edinburgh, Scotland.

Vogel, V. de, Ruiter, C. de, Beek, D. van, & Mead, G. (2004). Predictive validity of structural and actuarial risk assessment for sexual violence: A retrospective study in a Dutch sample of treated sex offenders. *Law and Human Behavior, 28*, 235-251.

Vijver, F.J.R. van de, & Leung, K. (1997). *Methods and data-analysis for cross-cultural research*. Thousands Oaks, CA: Sage.

Wallace, J.F., Schmitt, W.A., Vitale, J.E., & Newman, J.P. (2000). Experimental investigations of information-processing deficiencies in psychopaths: Implications for diagnosis and treatment. In C.B. Gacono (Ed.), *The clinical and forensic assessment of psychopathy: A practitioner's guide* (pp. 87-109). Mahwah, NJ: Erlbaum.

Wallace, J.F., Vitale, J.E., & Newman, J.P. (1999). Response modulation deficits: Implications for the diagnosis and treatment of psychopathy. *Journal of Cognitive Psychotherapy: An International Quarterly, 13*, 55-70.

Walters, G.D. (2003). Predicting institutional adjustment and recidivism with the Psychopathy Checklist Factor Scores: A meta-analysis. *Law and Human Behavior, 27*, 541-558.

Ward, T., McCormack, J., Hudson, S.M., & Polaschek, D. (1997). Rape: Assessment and treatment. In D.R. Laws & W. O'Donohue (Eds.), *Sexual deviance: Theory, assessment, and treatment* (pp. 356-393). New York: Guilford.

Webster, C.D., Douglas, K.S., Belfrage, H., & Link, B.G. (2000). Capturing change: An approach to managing violence and improving mental health. In S. Hodgins (Ed.), *Violence among the mentally ill: Effective treatment and management strategies* (119-144). Dordrecht, the Netherlands: Kluwer.

Webster, C.D., Douglas, K.S., Eaves, D., & Hart, S.D. (1997). *HCR-20: Assessing the risk of violence* (version 2). Burnaby, Canada: Mental Health, Law, and Policy Institute, Simon Fraser University.

Webster, C.D., Eaves, D., Douglas, K.S., & Wintrup, A. (1995). *The HCR-20 scheme: The assessment of dangerousness and risk*. Vancouver, Canada: Simon Fraser University and British Columbia Forensic Psychiatric Services Commission.

Webster, C.D., Harris, G.T., Rice, M.E., Cormier, C., & Quinsey, V.L. (1994). *The Violence Prediction Scheme: Assessing dangerousness in high risk men*. Toronto, Ontario, Canada: University of Toronto.

Weiler, B.L., & Widom, C.S. (1996). Psychopathy and violent behaviour in abused and neglected young adults. *Criminal Behaviour and Mental Health, 6,* 253-271.

Weiner, I.B. (1991). *Psychological disturbance in adolescence*. New York: Wiley.

Weiner, I.B. (1998). *Principles of Rorschach interpretation*. Mahwah, NJ: Erlbaum.

Weiner, I.B., & Exner, J.E. (1991). Rorschach changes in long-term and short-term psychotherapy. *Journal of Personality Assessment, 56,* 453-465.

Widiger, T.A., Cadoret, R., Hare, R.D., Robins, L.N., Rutherford, M.J., Zanarini, M., Alterman, A.I., Apple, M., Corbitt, E., Forth, A.E., Hart, S.D., Kultermann, J., & Woody, G. (1996). DSM-IV antisocial personality disorder field trial. *Journal of Abnormal Psychology, 105,* 3-16.

Widiger, T.A., & Corbitt, E.M. (1995). Antisocial personality disorder in DSM-IV. In J. Livesley (Ed.), *DSM-IV personality disorders* (pp. 127-134). New York: Guilford.

Widiger, T.A., Hurt, S.W., Frances, A., Clarkin, J.F., & Gilmore, M. (1984). Diagnostic efficiency and DSM-III. *Archives of General Psychiatry, 41,* 1005-1012.

Williamson, S., Harpur, T.J., & Hare, R.D. (1991). Abnormal processing of emotional words by psychopaths. *Psychophysiology*, *28*, 260-273.

Windle, M., & Dumenci, L. (1999). The factorial structure and construct validity of the Psychopathy Checklist-Revised (PCL-R) among alcoholic inpatients. *Structural Equation Modeling*, *6*, 372-393.

Wong, S. (1988). Is Hare's Psychopathy Checklist reliable without the interview. *Psychological Reports*, *62*, 931-934.

Wong, S. (1995). Recidivism and criminal career profiles of psychopaths: A longitudinal study. *Issues in Criminal and legal Psychology*, *24*, 147-152.

Wong, S. (2000). Psychopathic offenders. In S. Hodgins & R. Müller-Isberner (Eds.), *Violence, crime and mentally disordered offenders: Concepts and methods for effective treatment and prevention* (pp. 81-112). Chichester, UK: Wiley.

World Health Organzation (1992). *The ICD-10 classification of mental and behavioural disorders. Clinical description and diagnostic guidelines*. Geneva, Switzerland: Author.

Wulach, J. (1988). The criminal personality as a DSM-III-R antisocial, narcissistic, borderline, and histrionic personality disorder. *International Journal of Offender Therapy and Comparative Criminology*, *32*, 185-199.

Yalom, I.D. (1995). *The theory and practice of group psychotherapy* (4th ed.). New York: Basic .

Young (1994). *Cognitive therapy for personality disorders: A schema-focused approach*. Sarasota: Professional Resource Press.

Young, M., Justice, J., & Erdberg, P. (1999). Risk factors to violence among psychiatrically hospitalized forensic patients: A multimethod approach. *Assessment*, *6*, 243-258.

Zamble, E., & Quinsey, V.L. (1997). *The criminal recidivism process*. New York: Cambridge University Press.

Zimmerman, M. (1994). Diagnosing personality disorders. A review of issues and research methods. *Archives of General Psychiatry, 51*, 225-245.

Zimmerman, M., & Coryell, W.H. (1990). Diagnosing personality disorders in the community. *Archives of General Psychiatry, 47*, 527-531.

Zinger, I., & Forth, A.E. (1999). Psychopathy and Canadian criminal proceedings: The potential for human rights abuses. *Canadian Journal of Criminology, 40*, 237-276.

# CURRICULUM VITAE

Martin Hildebrand was born April 18th 1967 in Gouda, the Netherlands. He attended high school in Amersfoort from 1979 - 1986. In September 1986 he began his studies at the University of Maastricht. He obtained a "doctoraal" degree in health sciences (1993), and in law (1994). During his studies, he worked as a research assistant at the Academic Behavior Therapy Unit of the Community Mental Health Center of Maastricht (1991 - 1993).

In 1994 he began as a researcher at the Department of Law of Leiden University, in affiliation with the Netherlands Institute for the Studies of Crime and Law Enforcement (NISCALE), Leiden. In 1995 he resigned, and traveled in Australia and New Zealand.

In November 1996 he started working in the Dr. Henri van der Hoeven kliniek, a forensic psychiatric hospital in Utrecht, first as an assistant researcher and from 1998 as a research psychologist working on research on psychopathy.

Since June 2004 he is principal investigator at the Expertise centre for Forensic Psychiatry (EFP), Utrecht, the Netherlands. His areas of professional interest include criminal responsibility, personality assessment, psychopathy, and risk assessment — he is a (co-)translator of the Dutch versions of the *Sexual Violence Risk-20* (SVR-20), the Hare *Psychopathy Checklist-Revised* (PCL-R), and the *Historical Clinical Risk management-20* (HCR-20).

# LIST OF PUBLICATIONS

Arntz, A., **Hildebrand, M.**, & Hout, M. van den (1994). Overprediction of anxiety, and disconfirmatory processes, in anxiety disorders. *Behaviour Research & Therapy*, *32*, 709-722.

Derks, F.C.H., **Hildebrand, M.**, & Mulder, J. (1998). Forensische dagbehandeling: Resultaten in termen van psychosociaal welbevinden en recidive. [Forensic day-treatment: Results in terms of psychosocial well-being and recidivism]. *Tijdschrift voor Criminologie*, *40*, 273-287.

Dreessen, L., **Hildebrand, M.**, & Arntz, A. (1998). Patient-informant concordance on the structured clinical interview for DSM-III- disorders (SCID-II). *Journal of Personality Disorders*, *12*, 149-161.

**Hildebrand, M.**, & Ruiter, C. de (1998). Ontwikkelingen in het onderzoek naar psychopathie. [Developments in the research of psychopathy]. *De Psycholoog*, *7/8*, 314-320.

**Hildebrand, M.**, & Ruiter, C. de (1998). Verslag van de commissie wetenschappelijk onderzoek: De Nederlandse Rorschach databank en de Nederlandse normeringsstudie van het *Comprehensive System*. [The Dutch Rorschach database and normative study of the Comprehensive System]. *Nederlands Rorschach Tijdschrift*, *7*, 17.

**Hildebrand, M.**, & Ruiter, C. de (1999). Classificatie en diagnostiek bij forensisch psychiatrische patiënten. [Classification and assessment of forensic psychiatric patients]. In C. de Ruiter & M. Hildebrand (Red.), *Behandelingsstrategieën bij forensisch psychiatrische patiënten* (pp. 1-8). Houten, the Netherlands: Bohn Stafleu Van Loghum.

**Hildebrand, M.**, & Ruiter, C. de (1999). Een voorbeeld van een behandelsetting: De Dr. Henri van der Hoeven Kliniek. [An example of a treatment setting: The Dr. Henri van der Hoeven Kliniek]. In C. de Ruiter & M. Hildebrand (Red.), *Behandelingsstrategieën bij forensisch psychiatrische patiënten* (pp. 17-25). Houten, the Netherlands: Bohn Stafleu Van Loghum.

**Hildebrand, M.**, & Ruiter, C. de (1999). Response styles on the Rorschach and the MMPI-2. *Nederlands Rorschach Tijdschrift, 8*, 5-10.

**Hildebrand, M.**, & Ruiter, C. de (2000). Terbeschikkingstelling, recidive en risicotaxatie: De rol van psychopathie. [Treatment of forensic psychiatric patients, recidivism and risk assessment: The role of psychopathy]. *Delikt en Delinkwent, 30*, 764-774.

**Hildebrand, M.**, & Ruiter, C. de (2002). De Nederlandstalige versie van Hare's *Psychopathy Checklist-Revised*: Enige psychometrische bevindingen. [The Dutch version of Hare's *Psychopathy Checklist-Revised*: Some psychometric findings]. *Gedragstherapie, 35*, 329-339.

**Hildebrand, M.**, & Ruiter, C. de (2004). PCL-R psychopathy and its relation to DSM-IV Axis I and Axis II disorders in a sample of male forensic psychiatric patients in the Netherlands. *International Journal of Law and Psychiatry, 27*, 233-248.

**Hildebrand, M.**, & Ruiter, C. de (2004). Gestructureerde risicotaxatie: Een noodzakelijke bezigheid in de tbs. [Structured risk assessment: A necessity in the tbs-sector]. *Gedragstherapie, 37*, 55-59.

**Hildebrand, M.**, Ruiter, C. de, & Nijman, H. (2004). PCL-R psychopathy predicts disruptive behavior among male offenders in a Dutch forensic psychiatric hospital. *Journal of Interpersonal Violence, 19*, 13-29.

**Hildebrand, M.**, Ruiter, C. de, Vogel, V. de (2003). Recidive van verkrachters en aanranders na tbs: De relatie met psychopathie en seksuele deviatie. [Recidivism of rapists after tbs: The relation with psychopathy and sexual deviance]. *De Psycholoog, 38*, 114-124.

**Hildebrand, M.**, Ruiter, C. de, & Vogel, V. de (2004). Psychopathy and sexual deviance in treated rapists: Association with sexual and non-sexual recidivism. *Sexual Abuse: A Journal of Research and Treatment, 16*, 1-24.

**Hildebrand, M.**, Ruiter, C. de, Vogel, V. de, & Wolf, P. van der (2002). Reliability and factor structure of the Dutch language version of Hare's Psychopathy Checklist-Revised. *International Journal of Forensic Mental Health, 1*, 139-154.

Mersch, P.P.A., **Hildebrand, M.**, Hout, W.J.P. van, Lavy, E.H., & Wessel, I. (1992). Somatic symptoms in social phobia: A treatment method based on rational emotive therapy and paradoxical interventions. *Journal of Behavior Therapy and Experimental Psychiatry, 23*, 199-211.

Nijman, H., With, H-J. de, & **Hildebrand, M**. (2004). Meting van agressie onder tbs-gestelden. [Measuring of aggression of tbs-patients]. *Sancties*, 85-92.

Ruiter, C. de, & **Hildebrand, M**. (Red.) (1999). *Behandelingsstrategieën bij forensisch psychiatrische patiënten* [Treatment strategies for forensic psychiatric patients]. Houten, the Netherlands: Bohn Stafleu Van Loghum.

Ruiter, C. de, & **Hildebrand, M**. (2000). Recidiverisico bij seksuele delinquenten: De rol van psychopathie. [Risk of recidivism in sexual offenders: The role of psychopathy]. *Tijdschrift voor Criminologie, 42*, 214-231.

Ruiter, C. de, & **Hildebrand, M**. (2002). Over toerekeningsvatbaarheid. [About criminal responsibility]. In P.J. van Koppen, D.J. Hessing, H.F.M. Crombag, & H. Merkelbach (Red.), *Het recht van binnen: Psychologie van het recht* (pp. 687-697). Deventer, the Netherlands: Kluwer.

Ruiter, C. de., & **Hildebrand, M**. (2003). The dual nature of forensic psychiatric practice: Risk assessment and management under the Dutch TBS-order. In P.J. van Koppen & S.D. Penrod (Eds.), *Adversarial versus inquisitorial justice: Psychological perspectives on criminal justice systems* (pp. 91-106). New York: Kluwer/Plenum.

Vogel, V. de, & **Hildebrand, M**. (2001). De HCR-20: Een risicotaxatieschaal voor het beoordelen van het risico van gewelddadig gedrag. [The HCR-20: A risk assessment scale for the assessment of the risk of violent behavior]. *Gedragstherapie, 34*, 93-102.

Vogel, V. de, **Hildebrand, M**., Ruiter, C. de, & Derks, F. (2001). Transmuralisering en ambulantisering in de forensische psychiatrie. [Transmuralisation and ambulantisation in forensic psychiatry]. *Maandblad Geestelijke volksgezondheid, 56*, 780-794.

Vogel, V. de, Ruiter, C. de, **Hildebrand, M**., Bos, B., & Ven, P. van de (in press). Different ways of discharge and (risk of) recidivism measured by the HCR-20 and PCL-R in a sample of treated forensic psychiatric patients. *International Journal of Forensic Mental Health*.

Wessel, I., **Hildebrand, M.**, & Mersch, P.P.A. (1991). Sociale fobie: Een speurtocht naar de beste gedragstherapeutische behandeling. [Social phobia: A search for the best behavioral therapeutic treatment]. *De Psycholoog*, *9*, 385-390.


## TRANSLATIONS

**Hildebrand, M.**, Ruiter, C. de, & Beek, D.J. van (2001). *SVR-20: Richtlijnen voor het beoordelen van het risico van seksueel gewelddadig gedrag.* [SVR-20: Guidelines for the assessment of risk of sexual violence]. Utrecht, the Netherlands: Forum Educatief.

Philipse, M., Ruiter, C. de, **Hildebrand, M.**, & Bouman, Y. (2000). *HCR-20. Beoordelen van het risico van gewelddadig gedrag. Versie 2.* [HCR-20: Assessing the risk of violence (version 2)]. Nijmegen/Utrecht, the Netherlands: Prof.mr. W.P.J. Pompestichting/Dr. Henri van der Hoeven Stichting.

Vertommen, H., Verheul, R., Ruiter, C. de, & **Hildebrand, M**. (2002). *Handleiding bij de herziene versie van Hare's Psychopathie Checklist.* [Manual of the Dutch version of Hare's Psychopathy Checklist-Revised]. Lisse, the Netherlands: Swets Test Publishers.

Criminal Sciences backlist

J.A.C. Bevers et al.: An Independent Defence Before the International Criminal Court.
Proceedings of the Conference Held at The Hague, 1-2 November 1999 (2000)
ISBN 90 5170 514 X

M. Hildebrand: Psychopathy in the Treatment of Forensic Psychiatric Patients. Assessment,
Prevalence, Predictive Validty, and Clinical Implications (2004)
ISBN 90 3619 052 5

J.W. de Keijser: Punishment and Purpose. From Moral Theory to Punishment in Action
(2000) ISBN 90 5170 515 8

M. Malsch et al. (eds.): Complex Cases. Perspectives on The Netherlands Criminal Justice
System (1999) ISBN 90 5170 499 2

L. Meintjes – van der Walt: Expert Evidence in the Criminal Justice Process.
A Comparative Perspective (2001) ISBN 90 5170 528 X

J.F. Nijboer et al. (eds.): Harmonisation in Forensic Expertise. An Inquiry into the
Desirability of and Opportunities for International Standards (2000) ISBN 90 5170 498 4